# OXFORD
UNIVERSITY PRESS

Oxford University Press is a department of the University of Oxford. It furthers
the University's objective of excellence in research, scholarship, and education
by publishing worldwide. Oxford is a registered trade mark of Oxford University
Press in the UK and certain other countries.

Published in the United States of America by Oxford University Press
198 Madison Avenue, New York, NY 10016, United States of America.

Library of Congress Cataloging-in-Publication Data
Cole, Thomas R., 1949– author.
Title: Old man country : my search for meaning among the elders / Thomas R. Cole.
Description: New York : Oxford University Press, 2019.
Identifiers: LCCN 2019001345 | ISBN 9780190689988 (hardback)
Subjects: LCSH: Older men—United States. | Old age—United States. |
Aging—Social aspects—United States. | BISAC: PSYCHOLOGY / Social Psychology. |
PSYCHOLOGY / Developmental / Adulthood & Aging. | MEDICAL / Geriatrics.
Classification: LCC HQ1064.U5 C5265 2019 | DDC 305.26/10973—dc23
LC record available at https://lccn.loc.gov/2019001345

9 8 7 6 5 4 3 2

Printed by Sheridan Books, Inc., United States of America

*To my children,*
*Jake and Emma*

*And to my grandson,*
*Noah*

CONTENTS

## ACKNOWLEDGMENTS

I first thank the men who appear in this volume, who gave me their time and shared their lives with me in person, on the phone, and over Skype. It is not easy to be open about one's experience of deep old age, a time of life that our culture fears and denigrates. I also thank others who spoke with me and do not appear in the book: Eugene Buday, Stanislav Grof, Phil Hardberger, Keith Jackson, Robert Lane, Edmund Pellegrino, William J. Schull, and Rick Smith. I have taken the liberty of altering some individual quotes to make their meaning clearer to the reader. The sources for biographical, historical, and gerontological material in each chapter can be found in the Sources and Further Reading section.

I am most indebted to my friend and collaborator Ben Saxton. We began working together in 2009, when Ben was my research assistant while a graduate student in the English Department at Rice University. The best part of my workweek was the hour or two we spent thinking and discussing academic literature about aging, gender, and old men; getting to know each other; and sharing ideas and plans. Ben went on to a postdoctoral fellowship and then moved to New Orleans to begin researching and writing a book about poker. As we both moved away from purely academic work and supported each other's projects, Ben kept working as a research associate and colleague. When the seed for *Old Man Country* was planted, he helped water, fertilize, and nurture it. Every chapter bears the marks of his careful thoughts, editing and drafting suggestions, and support for a project that often seemed impossible or interminable.

Others helped me contact people I wanted to interview: Richard Buday, Bill Howze, Bob Goodrich, Emily Fine, Phil Montgomery, Rick Moody, Mark Ryan, John Schuster, and Steve Stein. I am grateful to others who spoke with me: Edie Beaujean, Susan Cooley, Elizabeth Coulter, Penelope Hall, Diane Highum, and Rick McCarthy. Sydney Callahan was especially generous in sharing her own experience as an old woman who has been Dan Callahan's wife for 65 years.

I am also indebted to many friends, colleagues, and others who made the book possible.

My agent, Beth Vesel, sought me out after reading a *New York Times* piece that quoted me. Over several years, she patiently but firmly shaped the proposal and the book itself. I am grateful to Abby Gross, my editor at Oxford University Press; Beth McLaughlin at Adept Word Management; and Andy Klein and David Kline for their research assistance and friendship.

My friends and colleagues in gerontology have saved me from many errors and brought new ideas as well as personal support for an unconventional project. Andy Achenbaum and I go back to the 1970s, when we were both graduate students in American history researching the nonexistent field of the history of aging. I am grateful for Andy's listening skills, wide-ranging knowledge, careful readings of draft chapters and above all, his friendship. Kate deMedeiros was my student at the Institute for Medical Humanities in Galveston in the 1990s. From the beginning, she provided input, fresh ideas about the dignity of all elders, and a sharp critical mind. Now a distinguished gerontologist, she has generously shared ideas, sources of data, gerontological literature, and her expertise in narrative gerontology.

My dear friend Marc Kaminsky has shaped this book in many ways: from early conversations about the arc, structure, and conception of the book to careful readings and unstinting support. Connie Royster has been my deep friend since middle school. She has listened to me talk about this book, offered suggestions, and made key connections for me. Catherine Stephenson has listened for many hours to the confusion and turmoil beneath the surface of the words written here. I am grateful for her interpretations, words of support and caution, and for moments of silence.

I am privileged to work as Director of the McGovern Center for Humanities and Ethics at The University of Texas Health Science Center At Houston. I am grateful to the center's faculty and staff colleagues—Nate Carlin, Rebecca Lunstroth, Angela Polczynski, and Alma Rosas—for their patience with and support for me these past several years. Alma efficiently helped organize the book's electronic files, facilitated transcriptions, helped research various questions, and gave her quiet support throughout what seemed like a never-ending process.

Finally, my wife Thelma Jean Goodrich has made this book possible. Her talents as a writer, her countless readings, her feminist angle of vision, her sensitivity as a psychotherapist, and her unstinting love, emotional support, and patience over many years are woven into every one of this book's pages.

| What My Fathers Couldn't Find

On September 22, 1953, my father, Burton David Michel, woke up early at our new house in New Haven, Connecticut. He turned over, kissed my mother, and wished her a happy 28th birthday. He came into my bedroom and kissed me. I was 4 years old. Next he kissed my brother and sister, 18-month-old twins sleeping in the next room. Then he dressed for work, ate breakfast, got into his brown four-door Packard, headed north on the Merritt Parkway, and drove his car into a bridge abutment.

I remember the phone ringing in the kitchen and our next-door neighbor, Mrs. Brownstein, rushing over. I remember the red and blue dots marking the white wrapping on the Wonder Bread waiting on the kitchen table. An ambulance took my father to a local hospital, where he lingered in a coma for a week. He never came home.

My mother seemed to disappear, too. She spent a week at his bedside, moved in with her parents for a while, and then went on a 2-week cruise with friends. My beautiful Aunt Carole came to stay with us.

It is said that everyone loved my father. People lined up around the block outside the funeral home for his funeral. The empty plot next to his grave at the Mishkan Israel Cemetery on Whalley Avenue still waits for my mother.

The family's version of my father's death is that it was an accident. Burt had been smoking, my grandmother said, and perhaps he lost control of the steering wheel. That story never made sense to me. It was a clear morning, there was no traffic on the highway, and the car crashed head-on.

In the late 1990s, Carole, still living in New Haven around the corner from my mother, was suffering from pancreatic cancer. My surgeon friend Steve Stein performed a "Whipple procedure" that extended her life. Just before the surgery, my aunt told Steve about a family secret that he thought

I should know, but he considered it a confidential element of their doctor–patient relationship. So he suggested that I do an oral history with Carole "to preserve her life story for the family."

When Carole got to her memories of my father's death, she hesitated.

"Oh, Tommy. . . . I'm so sorry . . . I don't want to hurt you."

"It's ok," I said. "I already know what you're going to say."

After the wreck, Carole spent several days keeping my mother company with the rest of the family gathered around my father's bed. After he died, a nurse gave Carole my father's belongings. In his wallet was a suicide note written for my mother. Carole tore up the note, flushed it down the toilet, and never spoke of it.

I never saw my mother cry or talk about my father's death. His pictures came down from the fireplace mantle. His Lehigh University fraternity mug and long sleek Sheaffer ink pen disappeared from the living room desk, along with every other trace of him.

One afternoon about a year after my father's death, I walked up the back-yard stairs into the screened-in porch at our house. A big strong man was sitting next to my mother on our green-and-white-webbed aluminum glider. Magically, he had fixed my bicycle. This big man's name was Bert Cole, and he was a veteran of World War II. I jumped into his lap. My mother married him soon afterward.

I had a long and difficult relationship with Bert Cole, who died in 2006 at the age of 88. Despite our struggles, I helped care for him at the end. I remember sitting one night in Room 452 of the Regional Hospital in Venice, Florida, watching him breathe as the clock silently witnessed our last time together, quieter and more serene than any before. That night, I slept on a sofa in his room. I was determined that my second father would not disappear like my first—without my being there.

The next morning, when my siblings and my mother arrived for the day's death watch, Bert's eyes were closed. His head hung to the left on the pillow, his slack mouth wide open—the look of the dying. No more use for the false teeth or glasses waiting on the nightstand. No more beeping from heart monitors or sounds of air whistling through breathing tubes. Only gurgling lungs and long irregular breaths disturbed the silence. As we watched over him, Bert suddenly woke up with a start, eyes wide as saucers. He looked around to see who was there—we three children and Jackie, all present and accounted for. Bert settled back against the pillow and closed his eyes. No one knew what he was thinking or what he understood. By turns, we talked to him, kissed him, and petted his head. He smiled and nodded each time. We contacted as many grandchildren as we could and held the phone up to his ear as each one spoke to him. He gestured and spoke toothlessly back. When my sister's daughter Sara spoke to him, he virtually shouted with joy, waving with his cold, bloated left hand. He spoke with his sister Sally. Then I suggested that we leave the room and give Jackie some private time to talk with him.

"I don't think I can do it," she sobbed.

"Of course you can," I said, taking her face between my hands and kissing her forehead.

After my mother talked to Bert, the four of us drove a few miles up Route 41 to Mi Pueblo for dinner. Halfway through the meal, the hospital nurse called: He was gone. I drove back to the hospital and sat with him until his body was taken to the morgue.

When I turned 60, I began reading and thinking seriously about becoming an old man myself. The following year, I underwent a difficult neck surgery to take pressure off peripheral nerves that were causing pain and weakness in my right arm. I began to read scholarly work about men and old age; memoirs and essays by old men (in particular Cicero, Malcolm Cowley, Donald Hall, and Roger Angell); and the fiction of Philip Roth, especially his slim novel *Everyman*. At the same time, I was watching popular films whose main characters were aging men played by Hollywood stars who were themselves aging—Harrison Ford, Sylvester Stallone, Clint Eastwood, and Tommy Lee Jones.

Most of all, I was captivated and haunted by the film adaptation of Cormac McCarthy's novel *No Country for Old Men*, whose main character, the aging Sheriff Ed Tom Bell, is faced with the overwhelming violence and terror of the Mexican drug trade. Set in a small Texas town, the movie is filled with bloody scenes of dead smugglers, mercenaries, and townspeople. But unlike the violent hypermasculine aging heroes in Westerns such as *Unforgiven* or *Cowboys and Aliens*, Sheriff Ed Tom Bell renounces violence and relinquishes the social scaffolding of middle-aged manhood. Faced with firepower that he cannot match and a kind of evil he cannot understand, Bell decides to retire. On a cold blustery day, he turns in his badge and walks out of the courthouse for the last time, the world utterly beyond his control. Bell sits in his truck for a few minutes, bitter and defeated. Like many aging men, Bell is no longer sure who he is or where he fits. He drives home to his wife Loretta to figure out what the next stage of his life will look like.

The film ends with a powerful dream. It is a cold snowy night. Bell is on horseback riding with his father through a mountain pass. His father moves on ahead and out of sight. Somewhere in the dark, he fixes a fire to warm and light his son's way. Bell knows that he will someday get to that place, and his father will be there. Then he wakes up.

Bell's dream has always moved me to tears. It evokes my longing for a father to light the way. As I write these words in April 2018, I am 69 years old. My mother is 93. My father would have been 92. My stepfather would have been 100. As I grow older, I continue to make peace with my father's suicide and with my stepfather's domineering and difficult personality. My first father, as my mother wrote on his gravestone, was "a man of tender conscience." He never found a way to live out his whole life. My second father lived into deep old age. He never found a way to share his life and love. He was, as my mother put it on *his* gravestone, "A Soldier to the End." In writing this book, I am looking for what my fathers couldn't find.

| Setting Out on Life's Journey

My father's death broke the sequence of generations in my four-year-old life. I was fated never to live out childhood's innocence or exuberance. But my father's death also sowed seeds of wisdom. Inside the darkness, I knew, like Ed Tom Bell, that somewhere on the path ahead there would be light.

When I was a young boy, the old people in my family were a sheltering rock. My grandparents and great aunts always seemed the same. They were there every weekend, on holidays, whenever we needed them. My brother, my sister, and I ate at their tables, roamed their houses, climbed in their yards, ravished their presents, and assumed their immortality.

My grandfathers died when I was 9 and 16 years old. My father's father Irving was a quiet, cigar-smoking blueprint shop owner who cried every day of his life after his son's death. The night Irving died, I had been on a local television show with my Cub Scout pack. My mother said he must have died happily after seeing me on TV. I wondered about that. My mother's father Jacob (known as Jack) was a hard-driving, self-made son of a Jewish immigrant tailor. Jack graduated from Yale University in 1912; his large, dark blue and white flannel Yale banner took up most of the wall over my brother's bed in our childhood bedroom. Jack's intensity, ambition, and success inspired and haunted me. I felt great pride at being a pallbearer at his funeral, where my uncontrollable crying disturbed an otherwise dignified affair.

My grandfathers were in their early 70s when they died. Their deaths were painful. But they didn't undermine the continuity derived from my grandmothers, who seemed to go on without change. Until my late 30s, they maintained their independence, each somewhat stern and difficult in her own way, each fiercely loyal and proud. Their existence helped frame my own. They demanded little and gave much.

In the spring of 1987, my mother's mother Helen entered the hospital for the first time since giving birth to my Aunt Carole. She died 2 weeks later. Helen was the family's matriarch. She possessed an upper-class bearing and an unwavering sense of dignity—as well as the wealth accumulated by Jack. She had always seemed invulnerable, as if she might actually outlive death, if not the rest of us. Her death was shocking despite her 87 years. It felt as if the rope of a great anchor had suddenly unraveled.

At age 85, my father's mother Reba, who was losing the ability to direct her own affairs, was forced out of the blueprint business she had run for 50 years. Her health was broken by cataracts and acute glaucoma, severe arthritis, stomach trouble, and, finally, Alzheimer's disease. In the fall of 1986, both Reba and my newborn daughter Emma were in diapers. Neither could walk more than a few steps without falling.

My grandmother fought furiously against me when, in the absence of my father, I had to take over her affairs and arrange a conservatorship and round-the-clock care for her. Reba had always been histrionic. "Keep this up and you'll kill your grandmother," she screamed at me across 2,000 miles of phone lines between Connecticut and Texas. "Is that what you want?" And then, after a long pause, she sighed. "Ah, but what can you do."

In 30 years, I would be having the same argument with my mother.

For 3 years, Reba stayed in her apartment with round-the-clock nursing care. At first, she tried to jump off her balcony and frequently hit or hollered at her caregivers, who once sent her to the emergency room in a straitjacket. After Reba had made several more traumatic visits to the hospital, I came to an understanding with her nurse's aides and physician: She would remain at home until she died. Reba had often expressed the wish for an end to her suffering, and we had recently decided against heroic measures to prolong her life. In 1988, she stopped walking altogether. Most of her time was spent sleeping or sitting in a wheelchair. Her legs contracted and curled up like chicken wings. Her skin broke down, and the sores became painful. Toward the end, she still had daily periods of lucidity.

One evening in late May 1989, Reba's caregivers telephoned. She had lost weight from vomiting and diarrhea, wasn't eating, and couldn't communicate. Would I give permission to insert an intravenous line for fluids and nutrition? I told them to keep feeding her with straws, bottles, or syringes and that we'd see how she was the next morning. After a guilt-ridden, sleepless night, I spoke to Beverly, who worked the day shift.

"Do you think she'd want an IV?" I asked.

"No, I don't think she'd want to be poked any more. Last week she said to me, 'Get out my blue dress and my shoes, because I'm going to die.'"

"OK," I said, my heart sinking. "Keep feeding her as much as she'll take by mouth, hold her, and tell her I love her." That day, Reba ate well and seemed to be rallying. She died the next morning, while Beverly and Geri were giving her a bath.

If only my father had lived. If only he had stayed with us and cared for his mother and my mother. If only he had stayed to take care of me and walk with me on the path of life.

Although I didn't realize it at first, my academic work as a historian, gerontologist, and professor of medical humanities has long been fueled by grief and by my search for guidance through the stages of life. Since the early 1980s, I've written and edited many books and produced films circling around the same questions: What does it mean to grow old? How do cultures weave the fabric of intergenerational relations to build meaningful lives? What is a good old age?

My thinking about aging has always been shaped by the image of life as a journey. In *The Journey of Life*—a book I wrote more than 25 years ago—I traced the history of cultural meanings of aging in Western Europe and the United States. I came to see that between antiquity and modernity, Western ideas about growing old changed dramatically. Aging was removed from the ancient provinces of religion and mystery and transferred to the modern terrain of science and mastery. Old age was removed from its place as a way station along life's spiritual journey and redefined as a problem to be solved by science and medicine.

If life is a journey, what shape does it take? Who accompanies us on the journey? How long does it last? Where does it begin and end? History and culture give us various answers. Sometimes, as the poet T. S. Eliot wrote in *Four Quartets*, the journey brings us full circle:

And the end of all our exploring
Will be to arrive where we started
And know the place for the first time.

Sometimes the journey appears as a kind of homecoming, as in Homer's ancient Greek epic poem the *Odyssey*. Odysseus, after fighting heroically in the Trojan War and confronting the Cyclops and other monsters, ultimately finds his way home to his wife Penelope. The hero's journey appeals to us when we realize that we too struggle against forces beyond our control. Worried and uncertain about how to confront our own monsters and find our direction, we remember that others share our struggle. In an interview for this book, the physician–writer Sherwin Nuland regretted that it took until his 70s to realize the importance of Philo of Alexandria's admonition: "Be kind, because everyone you meet is fighting a great battle."

The hero's journey takes the form of a fantastically popular religious allegory in 18th-century Englishman John Bunyan's *Pilgrim's Progress,* which charts Christian's solo journey from the City of Destruction to the Celestial City. The appeal of the journey from sin to salvation, of course, is the idea that God grants eternal life to a virtuous person. Like the hero in *Pilgrim's Progress,* American men tend to view the journey of life as an individual trip. We internalize the image of the self-made man who equates masculinity with independence and self-reliance and who thinks he can live as if middle age goes on forever. This way of thinking tends to view masculinity and femininity as polar opposites; it constrains our ability to accept dependence and the need for others.

Part II of *Pilgrim's Progress* follows Christiana, Christian's wife, as she travels with her children and her friend Mercy. Although Christiana's journey barely has a place in our cultural memory, her path remains the prevailing one for women, who more often accept the limitations of their bodies and feel the desire and need to travel with others. On my own travels to the elders while researching this book, I spoke with Sydney Callahan, Dan Callahan's wife, who put an unexpected twist on this pattern. "You've always had to deal with male privilege," she told me,

> And if you've been pregnant, which I have been seven times, you'd know what it's like to be physically limited and totally unable to do this or that, and you have to become dependent and interdependent. So women are trained at interdependence, and that's what I think is a great advantage.

How can men learn that dependence and interdependence are part of the journey? One way to begin is by acknowledging the fear, shame, and unhappiness we may feel because we inhabit bodies no longer as strong and conventionally beautiful as they once were. We can learn to accept and be compassionate toward our own declining body. The Irish poet William Butler Yeats struggled with these questions to the very end of his life. Yeats, who experimented with an early form of testosterone to maintain his vitality and sexual potency, also came to see the importance of spirituality. As he wrote,

> An aged man is but a paltry thing
> A tattered coat upon a stick, unless
> Soul clap and sing, and louder sing

For every tatter in its mortal dress.

What does it mean for "soul to clap and sing"? I think it can mean many things, from literally singing in a church choir to enjoying a sunrise, taking care of and playing with grandchildren, appreciating the gift of another day of life, being grateful for the presence and support of caregivers, gazing into the eyes of the love of one's life, and celebrating and working toward a future that extends beyond one's own life.

I often think of an old Jewish fable: *When each of us is born, an angel swoops down and slaps us on our bottom and whispers: "Grow!"* The problem is that most of us stop listening in midlife. We think there is no more growing to do. I believe that a good old age requires growth, which requires conscious effort and intention. It is an accomplishment made possible by social support, by favorable circumstances, and also by the love and care of others. *Old Man Country* is premised on the idea that however old we are, there is always a green growing edge in our story, always a hidden path of personal growth.

What do I mean by the terms "old" and "old age"? In truth, these words have multiple meanings and skirt any single definition. But history can help us understand these meanings and provide context for their usage today. Until the 18th century, most people in the West had little idea how "old" they were. Chronological age had little or no meaning in everyday life. Instead, people fell into a particular stage or "age" of life, based on their functioning and their place in family and community. The number of stages often varied. One scheme divided people into three ages: morning, noon, and evening. As in the ancient Greek riddle posed by the Sphinx to Oedipus: What goes on four legs in the morning, two legs at noon, and three legs in the evening? Answer: "man," who crawls on all fours at the beginning of life, stands upright in the middle of life, and walks with a cane in the last third of life.

In *As You Like It* (ca. 1600), Shakespeare revealed the theatrical origin of the metaphor of the "stages of life":

All the world's a stage.
And all the men and women merely players;
They have their exits and their entrances,
And one man in his time plays many parts,
His acts being seven ages.

In this scheme, the seven ages are infant, schoolboy, lover, soldier, justice, pantaloon, and old age. Many of us will remember the frightening words Shakespeare used to describe old age:

... Last scene of all,
That ends this strange eventful history,
Is second childishness and mere oblivion,
Sans teeth, sans eyes, sans taste, sans everything.

In some Western societies, the use of chronological age became possible as early as the 17th century, when church registers were developed to keep track of births, baptisms, marriages, and burials. Even then, a person's chronological age had little meaning in everyday life. In the 19th century, however, Western governments began using census data to track men for wartime purposes, chart the health of populations, and create a uniform age for retirement benefits in what became the welfare state. By the 20th century, Western countries used chronological age to channel people bureaucratically into the three boxes of life: school, work, and retirement. As mass longevity became a reality in many areas of the world, "old age" was of little use in describing people who could range in age from 55 to 100 years. Gerontologists introduced the concepts of "young old," "old old," and "oldest old."

The last quarter of the 20th century saw a new awareness and encouragement of the youthfulness, health, and well-being of our aging population. Since then, a new version of the "ages" or "stages" model of the life course has appeared in scientific thinking and popular culture. In 1989, Peter Laslett's book, *A Fresh Map of Life: The Emergence of the Third Age*, drew attention to masses of people who were retired, in reasonable health, well-educated, and living without any prescribed direction or activity (except the pressures of consumerism and remaining youthful). Laslett named that period of life—between the completion of careers and child-rearing and the onset of frailty—the Third Age. That name helped spawn an educational movement known as Universities of the Third Age in Europe, which paralleled the growth of Institutes for Learning in Retirement in the United States, along with movements for conscious aging, positive aging, successful aging, and sacred aging—all self-conscious ways of helping older people live more engaged and fulfilled lives. The concept of the Third Age corresponded to a sea change in perceptions of the possibilities and prospects of the Baby Boom generation (76 million born 1946 and 1964), which began turning age 65 in 2011.

Due to improved nutrition, public health measures, and medical care, Americans generally live much healthier and longer lives than ever before, although longevity is not distributed equally across race or class and is even declining is some areas. In 1900, the average American man lived to age 47, and the average woman lived to age 49. In 2017, the average American man lived to age 79, and the average woman lived to age 81. Unfortunately, growing numbers of older people are financially vulnerable or falling into poverty due to the fraying of the welfare state and inadequate savings and pension plans.

Today, 10,000 Americans turn age 65 years every day; the average man who turns age 65 can expect to live to approximately age 85 and the average woman to age 87. What we usually fail to notice is the aging of the aging population, or the "Fourth Age"—a stage of life roughly demarcated by age 80 or older. Today, the number of people age 80 or older in the United States is growing twice as fast as those older than age 65 and almost four times the growth rate of the total US population. The Fourth Age is often—but not always—marked by increasing frailty; declining ability for self-care; and vulnerability to disease, disability, and dependence. And, of course, it always ends in death. The Fourth Age has been described as a Black Hole—a vague, frightening, and shadowy cultural space that evokes denial when it doesn't provoke fear. In one sense, the Fourth Age today marks a return of Shakespeare's characterization of old age, the last stage of life, as "second childishness and mere oblivion." But the Fourth Age also contains periods of sheer fun, appreciation of beauty, powerful religious and/or spiritual experience, community and family engagement, and continued work and artistic development.

*Old Man Country* seeks to reclaim and enhance the humanity of men in the Fourth Age. (I seek, of course, to reclaim and enhance the humanity of old women as well. That is another project, well underway thanks to scholars, activists, artists, and the sheer force of example.) To learn more about men in the Fourth Age, I decided to talk to those who were living it. It is a strategy first made famous in Plato's *Republic,* in which Socrates says to Cephalus,

> There is nothing which for my part I like better, Cephalus, than conversing with aged men; for I regard them as travellers who have gone on a journey which I too may have to go, and of whom I ought to enquire, whether the way is smooth and easy, or rugged and difficult.

To begin, I made a list of men I admired and wanted to talk to. I asked friends for advice. Many people on my list declined, couldn't be reached, or never responded to my inquiry. I couldn't reach my childhood folk song hero Pete Seeger, on whose banjo were inscribed the words "This machine surrounds hate and forces it to surrender." Pete died in 2014 at age 94. Bill Moyers, former Press Secretary for President Lyndon Johnson and longtime public television host and documentary film-maker, responded that he had too much work to do and hadn't given it much thought. Sidney Poitier's agent told me that he was too busy working in civil rights and the struggle against racism. The novelist Philip Roth, who died in May 2018, never responded to my letters. I did reach the famed, longtime ABC sportscaster Keith Jackson, and we spoke by phone. When I asked what he looked forward to, he answered, "tomorrow."

I was never able to contact the wise and melancholy singer–songwriter Leonard Cohen, whose song "Anthem" contains a verse stored deep in my spiritual rolodex:

> Ring the bells that still can ring
> Forget your perfect offering.
> There is a crack in everything.
> That's how the light gets in.

Some conversations took place but never made it into the book. Of these, the saddest and most vivid was my encounter with 99-year-old Robert Lane, a former Yale University political scientist and activist. Tortured by an untold past filled with pain and regret, Lane was weary of life when I met him at an assisted living facility in New Haven, Connecticut. Drool steadily slid off his chin and painted brown spots on his tan jacket as he poured his heart out to me. "You are like a therapist," he said to me after 2 hours. Lane then spent a sleepless night horrified that his inner life might be made public. The next day, he contacted me in anger and revoked the written permission he'd given me to use the transcripts of the interview.

*Old Man Country* explores how 12 men face (or faced) the challenges of living a good old age. All who appear in this volume are highly accomplished. Some are friends. Some are strangers. Some are famous: Paul Volcker, the former head of the Federal Reserve under Presidents Reagan and Carter; Hugh Downs, veteran TV broadcaster and creator of "The Today Show"; Denton Cooley, the first surgeon to implant an artificial heart into a human being; and Ram Dass, his generation's foremost American teacher of Eastern spirituality.

Others are less famous but no less accomplished. George Vaillant is a research psychiatrist who directed the pre-eminent longitudinal study of elite American men from their college years until death. Red Duke was a trauma surgeon who founded the nation's second (and now busiest) life-flight helicopter service. Sherwin Nuland was a physician–writer best known for *How We Die*, which won the National Book Award in 1994. John Harper is a former English professor from the University of Iowa who came out as gay when it was dangerous to do so and has made countless contributions to the intellectual, social, and cultural life of Iowans. Sam Karff is one of the great rabbis of his era. James Forbes is a powerful preacher who served as the first African American Senior Minister at Riverside Church in Manhattan. Dan Callahan is co-founder of The Hastings Center, an independent think tank that studies key issues in bioethics and life sciences. Walter Wink was a radical Christian theologian, writer, and activist who was in the late stages of Lewy body dementia when we talked in 2011.

All of these men, when I talked to them, were in their 80s and 90s—in or verging on the Fourth Age. They were born long before feminism began to challenge male dominance and civil rights movements began to fight for the rights of African Americans and gay, lesbian, transgender, queer, and disabled persons. In addition to male privilege, most of these men also enjoy the advantages of being white, Protestant, heterosexual, and financially comfortable. Their privileged status, however, did not guarantee their success. Nor has it exempted them from suffering and loss. Several have become frail and in need of assistance since I talked with them. Some have lost partners. Others have died.

My interviews were not structured by the methodology of social science, conducted by asking identical questions, recording the answers, and categorizing and analyzing them. They were often highly personal conversations, aimed at a mutual listening and telling in which we might both learn something new about ourselves. I was more interested in their current experience than in their earlier accomplishments. Sometimes, the conversations simply flowed from an opening gambit: "So, how is your life now that you are old?" Sometimes I asked the following questions, although not in any particular order:

How did you spend the day yesterday? Do you have a daily routine?
What do you love? Whom do you love? What is the role of sexuality in your life?
What do you look forward to?
What are you afraid of?
What were the high points of your life? The low points?
How do you think about your legacy?
What do you regret? What would you do differently if given the chance?
What does it mean to be an old man? A man?
What should old men be contributing to the world today?

As I talked with these men, four major challenges or questions kept surfacing: (1) Am I still a man? (2) Do I still matter? (3) What is the meaning of my life? and (4) Am I still loved? Each man's identity is bound up with all these questions. Because the boundaries of these questions are porous, the answer to one is also part of the answer to another. I have separated them here for the sake of clarity and to organize the book into four corresponding sections.

## Am I Still a Man?

Masculinity is not a natural collection of individual traits but, rather, a cultural story, a plot, or a script by which men are judged and judge themselves. In the United States, the dominant story of masculinity is still that of the self-made man who proves himself at school, in sports, in the military, in business, in politics—in every competitive arena of a market-based society. Physical strength, self-control, aggression, and competitiveness are hallmarks of this story of masculinity.

One problem is that this script for masculinity stops at midlife. We lack guidelines for "being a man" in the Third Age and especially the Fourth Age, limiting our ability to fashion culturally effective identities. For most old men in American society, there are no landmarks of achievement or value; no lighthouse guiding one's moral compass; no employment office with the sign "old men wanted." There is only the province of retirement—a barren place, often marked by an absence of wealth, prestige, and personal meaning.

When the men discussed in this book were growing up, a particularly elitist model of self-reliant manhood prevailed in American culture. In 1963, sociologist Erving Goffman outlined the benchmarks of this largely unstated model: "There is only one complete unblushing male in America," he wrote. That male was

> young, married, white, urban, northern, heterosexual, Protestant, father of college education, fully employed, of good complexion, weight and height, and a recent record in sports. . . . Any male who fails to qualify in any one of these ways is likely to view himself—during moments at least—as unworthy, incomplete, and inferior.

Except for George Vaillant and Paul Volcker, most of the men discussed in this book could never fully enter this exclusive club. As an African American and Southerner, Reverend James Forbes would be ruled out in advance, as would John Harper, a gay man from rural Iowa. The rugged trauma surgeon from Texas, Dr. Red Duke, would likely have laughed at the idea that he needed to measure up to a Yankee ideal. Dan Callahan is a Catholic, Sherwin Nuland and Sam Karff are Jews, Wink is another Texan, and so on. And in growing old, each of these men also literally outlived the youthful model of American masculinity.

How do men meet the challenge of reconciling manhood with physical decline? There is no single way. One is to reject the model altogether, integrating traditionally "female" traits of caring, acknowledging emotion, and valuing relationships. George Vaillant articulates this path and focuses on creativity rather than masculinity. On the other hand, for physician–writer Sherwin Nuland, who died in 2014, maintaining manhood meant continuing to write and remaining strong by working out at the gym. Reverend Dr. James Forbes faces it as a Christian man committed to his faith and to the struggle against racism. John Harper feels somewhat diminished because he can no longer have orgasms. For some, the problem of masculinity— including the loss of sexual potency—disappears in old age: Dan Callahan thinks of himself as a person, not as a man.

## Do I Still Matter?

In 1922, psychologist G. Stanley Hall, who had recently retired as President of Clark University, published *Senescence*—a gloomy book that virtually invented the field of gerontology. Feeling isolated and irrelevant in his transition "from leadership to the chimney corner," Hall envisioned a time when "graybeards" would find renewed moral authority and social purpose. "The chief thesis of this book," he wrote, "is that we have a function in this world that we have not yet risen to and which is of utmost importance." If Hall's comments were prescient about the plight of old men, they were overly optimistic about its solutions.

In the late 1960s, psychiatrist Robert Butler coined a term that encapsulates the devaluation of both older men and women in American society. *Ageism*, he pointed out, is a deep cultural prejudice toward old people manifested in stereotypes, myths, assumptions, and discrimination. Although the media and consumer culture present many positive images of old people remaining young, these images also contain another form of ageism, barely disguising the fear and loathing in store for old people who can no longer look youthful, perform midlife roles, and maintain their independence. We have precious few images of dignity in deep old age or independence.

It is safe to say that old men—even those who have preserved their youthfulness—have yet to find a function of "utmost importance" or even of much importance at all. At least since the institutionalization of retirement in the mid-20th century, aging and old men have often felt marginalized, useless, or invisible. Retirement is a primary source of depression for those whose identities and self-esteem have depended on being productive, earning a living, and being engaged with others in the workplace. Today, approximately 20% (this number has crept up in recent years) of men older than age 65 are working part- or full-time. After retirement, approximately one-fourth of men perform some form of volunteer work in their communities.

Employment and volunteer work are often less possible for men who have reached their 80s. When a man is frail or dependent on others to carry out the activities of daily life, the question "Do I still matter?" becomes even more pressing. The challenge of being relevant is the challenge of learning and creating new things, being engaged with others. making a difference in the lives of other people, being committed to a future beyond oneself, and feeling needed.

For some people, being needed means greeting people at hospitals, bringing meals to old people who can't leave their homes, or taking care of grandchildren. For Paul Volcker, retired Chairman of the Federal Reserve, "being needed" means being at or close to the center of power and decision-making authority. Despite his age and apparent irrelevance during the financial crisis of 2008, Volcker convinced the Obama administration to implement what became "the Volcker Rule," limiting banks' ability to make risky investments with ordinary peoples' savings accounts. Volcker continues to feel obligated to contribute his gifts and skills. When I talked to him, he had new ideas for professional education in public administration. But he couldn't convince schools or donors to establish new programs.

Among the other men to whom I talked, the question "Do I Still Matter?" was particularly bound up with work. Even after writing or editing 47 books over more than 50 years, Dan Callahan's identity still depended on his next article or book. When we spoke, Dan was feeling no incentive or energy to write—an emotional and existential crisis for him.

Sam Karff, after retiring as a congregational rabbi, worked half-time for 12 years helping medical students become more compassionate. At age 86, he remains active in community life, continues to write, and studies his biblical spiritual texts. He also enjoys his daily naps at an assisted living facility.

Each man finds forms of engagement consistent with his personal history. Hugh Downs was still driving, studying physics, traveling, and appearing on television shows at age 93. For heart surgeon Denton Cooley, who died 3 years after I interviewed him in 2013, relevance took the forms of going to the office every day, managing his money, and burnishing his legacy. John Harper was long retired both from the English Department at the University of Iowa and from the Episcopal Church when I talked to him. Yet he was still trying to finish a history of the English Department at the University of Iowa and performing religious ceremonies at his church. That night he was scheduled for rehearsal at the local community theater he had founded.

In my view, we must build a country where all men, and women, matter in the Fourth Age; where we are valued as elders who contribute to society but are not demeaned if we become ill and dependent; where we are free to run marathons but do not feel like failures for slowing down; where we work to maintain health but can find dignity in frailty; where we feel free to climb mountains and also to ponder the meaning of our lives; where excessive emphasis on health and activity does not crowd out time to think about what really matters; where humane care of the dying takes precedence over futile, expensive, high-tech interventions at the end of life; and where death and dying can be viewed as the culmination of a well-lived life.

## What Is the Meaning of My Life?

If modern society lengthened old age, it also drained it of cultural meaning— a feature of secularization first noted in the 1960s when Swiss physician A. L. Vischer wondered "whether there is any sense, any vital meaning in old age." In the same vein, psychoanalyst Erik Erikson drew the conclusion that because we lack a viable ideal of late life, "our civilization does not really harbor a concept of the whole of life."

Because our society provides old people with no widely shared meanings or norms by which to live, the task of finding significance in later life falls to individuals in their relationships with family and community.

Meaning is partly a matter of love and of relevance. If I love and am loved, my life has significance. If I have family, friends, community, or good caregivers, my life matters because it matters to them and because I am committed to them. Meaning is also a moral question: Have I lived a good life by my own lights? Did I, and do I, measure up to my own expectations and to the standards of my family, religion, community, and nation?

Learning to feel at home in old age means believing that our life matters even in the face of frailty, disease, and death. A central developmental task here is the paradoxical work of learning to hold on and let go—working, on the one hand, to stay healthy, to care for ourselves and others; and learning to discern, on the other hand, when it is time to accept that we really do need help from others or when it is time to let go of life. Learning to find meaning on both sides of this paradox is the spiritual work of aging. It is not work that our culture encourages.

What does my life mean? For many people, existential meaning derives from living inside religious, spiritual, or philosophical traditions whose ideas, symbols, and rituals point us toward some form of transcendence, often assumed to be "the" ultimate truth. Reverend James Forbes's life revolves around a Christian love inspired by the life of Jesus, infused with the struggle for social justice, and filled with the grace of the Holy Spirit. When I met Hugh Downs at age 93, I learned that this world-famous television broadcaster is immersed in contemporary physics and finds personal meaning in a benevolent universe that runs according to the laws of nature. Sam Karff believes in a personal God and finds meaning in the tradition of rabbinic storytelling and in fulfilling the ethical commandments inherent in the Covenant.

Another answer to the question of meaning comes from affirming that we are each links in a chain of generations. We find strength by looking back to our ancestors and forward to our descendants. I have always been pained by the generational link broken by my father's suicide. But today, my face turns more toward future generations than past generations. Just recently, my daughter Emma gave birth to a baby boy—my grandson, Noah Cole Hillson. Noah is a new link in the chain. His life strengthens mine and changes my place in our family story. I can't wait to know him as he grows up, celebrate his life, help care for him, and support his future. Within the past year, my sister's daughters have had daughters of their own. The meaning of my aging is bound up with their futures as well.

For those men without children, commitment to a future beyond their own lives comes in many forms: teaching, caregiving, community life, environmental and political advocacy, and spiritual growth that leads to self-transcendence. John Harper, for example, has spent what seems like a lifetime engaged in community theater, gay activism, university teaching, and the building of progressive church communities in Iowa City.

## Am I Still Loved?

Love, of course, means many things. There is love of God, for example—a commandment in Judaism that Sam Karff tries to live by acting justly, mercifully, and humbly. There is also love that *comes* from God or a Divine Being or Beings—love that carries existential meaning. This is the kind of love that Walter Wink had in mind when he told his wife June that he wanted to go "home to Jesus." It is the kind of love Ram Dass received from his guru Neem Karoli Baba, who inspired him to live a life of loving service on the path toward merging with Brahman, the ultimate reality in Hinduism.

I have never been able to feel personally loved by a traditional God. I do, however, believe in an unknowable transcendent force that can be glimpsed through religious stories, symbols, images, and religious lenses. This perspective first became clear to me when my 13-year-old daughter Emma came home from religious school one day. "Dad, I don't believe in God," she said. "It's just a story." "Yes," I said, "But it's a very special story." In prayer or meditation, when I imagine God as the Creator who fashioned me as part of his or her ongoing creation of the world, I sometimes feel embraced by a benevolent presence. I must admit that I am envious of people who do feel that God loves them, as in the powerful lyrics from the song "Outrageous" by Paul Simon, who asked in his 60s,

> Who's gonna love you when your looks are gone?
> Yea, who's gonna love you when your looks are gone?
> God will.
> Just like he waters the flowers at your window sill.

Love also comes in the forms of friendship, family or caregiving relationships, or the less personal form of loving strangers or other living beings. Such love makes us who we are. Long-time loving friends, for example, preserve memories and identities. When we lose a friend from childhood, we lose a deep and elemental part of ourselves. Memories disappear: No one else will remember you as a sixth grader or your humiliation at being fired as a grammar school crossing guard because you were listening to a Yankees game on your transistor radio. You are only a father or uncle because of your children, nieces, and nephews, and you are only a grandfather because of your grandchildren. The strength of those identities rests on the strength of their constitutive relationships and on efforts to keep love from being overshadowed by the inevitable darker emotions such as resentment and anger. Feeling your connection to the natural world can also be a source of love.

Most often, we think about erotic or romantic love, which plays a more or less salient role in the lives of almost all these men. Historically, love has been the cultural prerogative of the young; love in later life has most often been mocked or derided, as in the image of the "dirty old man" or the old woman who refuses to "act her age" and hide her desire. Until the late 20th century, sex in old age was taboo. Since then, sexuality and erotic love among old people have come out of the closet.

George Vaillant recently summarized a key finding of his research on men over a lifetime: "Happiness is only the cart. Love is the horse." His central point is that maintaining long-term loving relationships with partners, family, friends, and in community is essential to a good old age. But in order to be fulfilled by love, "You have to be able to take it in," he says, "You have to feel inside that you are loved." In addition, love and connection add significantly to longevity and overall health.

Dan Callahan has been married to Sydney Callahan for 65 years. In our conversation, she dampened expressions of love for him out of deference to his unemotional personal style. He is deeply in love with and dependent on her, although I had to pull teeth to get him to talk about their relationship. To the very end of his life, Walter Wink alternated between resisting and accommodating dementia. Both were made possible because his wife June was there to love and care for him daily.

*Old Man Country* aims to help men—and the women, children, relatives, friends, and lovers around them—become more conscious of their own aging, to grow into the last stage of life with awareness and the courage to face the four challenges of the Fourth Age: masculinity, relevance, meaning, and love. Each man faces these challenges in his own way, guided by his culture, located in his family and community, and constrained by the circumstances of his life history. Each man is everyman, and each man is his own unique self. So it is with all of us. If we want to anchor our own identities and become citizens worthy of the country we are hoping to build, we too will need to grapple with these questions.

*Old Man Country* is also a personal book. Each chapter tells a story of my conversation with an elder, including my observations, insights, reactions, and feelings. Set alongside stories of these encounters, you will find interludes, key moments from my own life story. In these, you will read about me as a small boy, as someone who grows up, and as someone who is now growing old. In a sense, the book is an autobiographical field report, a memoir of my own journey toward an uncertain wisdom, and the final payment on my childhood's psychic debt.

PART I | Am I Still a Man?

| George Vaillant and the Good Life of the American Man

Early one clear morning, I fly into John Wayne Airport in Orange, California, rent a little blue Dodge Dart, check into my hotel room in Santa Anna, and drive for 30 minutes to meet George Vaillant. I am surprised to find his modest house perched up on a small hill just off a busy four-lane highway. It's a far cry from the Ivy-covered walls of Harvard University and the colonial wooden or Victorian brick homes in Cambridge, Massachusetts. Vaillant comes out to meet me in khaki shorts, a short-sleeved polo shirt, and sockless rubber-soled docksiders. Even now, he has the air of a Harvard professor who smokes a pipe and wears tweed jackets with leather elbow patches.

"George Vaillant," he says, extending his hand.

Vaillant probably knows more than anyone else about what it takes to be a successful old man in American culture. Or rather, he knows more about what did or did not lead to a good old age for the 268 Harvard men who participated in the Grant Study—a research project that began in 1937 and continues to this day. Vaillant, who was 4 years old when the study began, became its research director in 1967. For more than 75 years, 268 of these elite exemplars of American masculinity (they include Ben Bradlee, long-time editor of the *Washington Post*, and President John F. Kennedy) regularly submitted to medical exams, gave interviews, filled out questionnaires, and took psychological tests. Their privileged place in society is reflected in their longevity. Whereas only 3% of the white male population born in 1920 survived to age 90, at least one-fourth of the Grant Study men were still alive and in their 90s when Vaillant published his most recent book, *Triumphs of Experience: The Men of the Harvard Grant Study* in 2012. Still, these men were not immune from life's hardships: By age 50, one-third of them met Vaillant's criteria for mental illness at one time or another.

At the outset of the study, these men epitomized the dominant image of young white Anglo-Saxon Protestant (WASP) northern masculinity that reigned in America throughout most of the 20th century. Vaillant is both an exemplar and a scholar of traditional WASP manhood, which excludes old men by definition. When he took over the Grant Study at age 33, the Harvard psychiatrist began with this same ageist prejudice that he would later fight so hard against. "After a man reached 50, I thought it was downhill all the way," he says, remembering his early assumptions, "and I was going to chart that." Vaillant's first application to the National Institute on Aging for funding to continue the study was rejected. The great gerontologist Jim Birren, who was 70 years old at the time, told Vaillant that he could not define aging in terms of decay alone. Aging, he instructed the 50-year-old Vaillant, was a vital life process, not a process of biological senescence to be postponed as long as possible. Still, even a decade into the study, Vaillant remembers that he was "scared stiff of everything after 65." These comments were a far cry from the man known today for championing the positive aspects of growing old.

When Vaillant was in his 30s and 40s, he thought in black-and-white categories. His goal in the Grant Study was to predict "good and bad outcomes." He assumed that the pathways to health and well-being in later life would conform to clear patterns of individual success in love and work. Pathways to unhappiness would be predicted by alcoholism, faulty coping mechanisms, and divorce. Over the course of the study, a man named Charles Boatwright disrupted Vaillant's rigid categories. Based on his life history, Boatwright had every reason to be miserable. His father was manic–depressive, difficult, and often cruel to his son. His marriage of 30 years was falling apart. His work history was checkered, including a long period of discontent in the corporate world. "He seemed to me occupationally feck-less," wrote Vaillant. "At that point in my life I didn't see much to exemplify optimum adult development at that point in his, and I let him slide gently off my radar."

But something strange happened. In 2009, when Boatwright was 89 years old, Vaillaint's colleague Monika Ardelt told him that Boatwright scored higher on her wisdom scale than any other man in the study. At age 49, Boatwright completed a questionnaire that seemed to belie his life experience. "I feel a marked change has come over me," he wrote,

> I have learned to be more kind and have more empathy. I have learned to be tolerant. I have a much better understanding of life, its meaning and purposes.

I've left the church, but in many ways I feel more Christian. I now understand . . . the old, the meek, the hard worker, and most of all children.

When 75-year-old Vaillant took another look, he realized that Boatwright's positive outlook and maturity had eluded the Grant Study's academic categories and developmental tasks. "I recognized that it wasn't he who had suddenly matured," Vaillant wrote. "It was I. I had finally learned that hope and optimism are not emotions to be dismissed lightly; perhaps this was a reflection of some spiritual growth of my own."

Boatwright also transcended the individualistic expectations built into the Harvard model of manhood. He *had* actually made a career. It was a career, as Vaillant put it, of "looking after others needier than himself." After leaving a stultifying corporate life, Boatwright moved to Vermont, where he helped build a lumber cooperative, a farmers' cooperative, an egg cooperative, and a high school. He volunteered as town auditor in Stowe, Vermont, and at age 89 was still exercising and volunteering 3 hours a week. Boatwright lived with his first wife (and didn't reveal her alcoholism) until she fell in love with an old friend and left the marriage. He then found a new and deeper love, which Vaillant notes is by far the most powerful predictor of a flourishing life. "No one has ever healed me with such love," Boatwright said of his second wife, "We have been enormously happy." Contrary to the dominant mold of masculinity, Boatwright didn't conform to expectations of a man's linear lucrative career and a single long-lived marriage.

I have admired Vaillant's research and writing from a distance for many years, amazed at the range of his interests and his unique combination of psychoanalytic, quantitative, and literary abilities. But now, as I sit at his dining room table, I want to talk about experience rather than knowledge. In particular, I wonder how it feels to be old and whether he feels less complete as a man.

I ask him, "Do you think of yourself as an old man now? What does it feel like?"

"Oh, I'm very happy," he says and immediately shifts to the intellectual: "You know what Jung said when someone was talking to him about how it felt to be 80? He said, I'm quoting loosely here, 'I am old, so I be's old. I'm not a bloody American.'"

"How old are you, chronologically speaking?"

"I'm 79.4."

"So you haven't exactly crossed the threshold into old age. But do you think of yourself as old?"

"Yeah, there is no question about it," he says, pivoting back to intellectual matters. "I mean, it is very clear that my last book was the last one I would write, that Sophocles could go on until 90, but it gets harder to write books."

Vaillant recently retired from Harvard and moved to Orange, California, to follow Dr. Diane Highum—his fourth wife, also a psychiatrist. The transition has not been easy.

"So what do you do when you get up in the morning?"

"I go upstairs, I check my email, and then I work on whatever writing I'm doing."

"Do you have a routine?"

"Yeah. No, no. I mean . . . my model for growing old is Churchill, who won the Nobel Prize for Literature at age 79," says Valliant. "When you ask, 'What did I do yesterday?' the first answer that comes to my mind is, 'I don't remember.' It's not worth your time to let me associate to get that."

"Yes it is. Yes, it is," I answer. "That's exactly what I'm interested in—your ordinary life. I'm interested in what you did yesterday or this morning."

I went for a walk yesterday. I'm writing a paper on positive psychiatry, and I spent the day going through various things I've written and trying to cobble them together. Now I read a lot but I don't remember it. And so what I can do creatively is what Sherrington did when someone said, "Professor Sherrington, you don't read the literature," and he said, "Of course I don't read the literature. I *am* the literature." That's the sign of an old man.

I smile at the wit of this remark, which moves surreptitiously from daily life to an academic anecdote. Funny but evasive. So I decide to ask him a more direct question: "What is the role of sexuality in your life?"

"Zero," he says without missing a beat. "When I was 75 I became impotent, and I never had been impotent before, and I chalked it up to what happens in most people's lives somewhere between 65 and 90, and for me it was 75."

"Is manhood separable from sexuality?" I ask.

Oh, it's totally separable. . . . The idea of not being able to penetrate is sad for my wife, but . . . it's one thing I can't do. To me creativity is so much more important than sexuality, and the fact is that I've been lucky enough to be creative. I have put things in the world that weren't there before, including my children and my writing.

A few minutes later, Vaillant's wife Diane comes home from work. Recovering from a serious foot injury, she rolls herself into the room, one knee leaning on what looks like an elevated skateboard propelled by her other leg. Diane, 15 years his junior, works at the University of California Irvine Medical Center. When she sits down at the table and smiles at me, I can see that I have an ally. Diane also wants George to speak from experience rather than from intellect. When she joins the conversation, things get more complicated.

"Tell me what you are afraid of," I say to him.

"Maybe you should ask me," she laughs.

After joking that he's not afraid of anything, Vaillant acknowledges that he *is* afraid of novelty and that moving to Orange from Cambridge was "scary." Then he shifts the focus to a global level: "I mean, if I say . . . what are the catastrophes I can see happening, overpopulation and destruction of the planet by sheer Darwinian—"

"But that's intellectualization," Diane interrupts. "He's talking about what you are personally afraid of."

"You can say what I'm afraid of, darling," George replies sarcastically.

"Loss of control," Diane responds immediately.

Their bantering makes me uncomfortable, so I shift ground. "What are the low points and the high points of your life?"

"This is one of the high points right here," he smiles and says, pointing to Diane. They met 6 or 7 years ago at an American Psychiatric Association meeting where George spoke about how faith, hope, and love were absent from the discourse of psychiatry.

"And the lowest point of my life," he says, "was probably when my father killed himself."

I am stunned. "My father killed himself, too," I blurt out.

"Really?" says Vaillant. "How old were you?"

I put up four fingers.

Vaillant was 10 years old when his father, George Clapp Vaillant, Sr., then drinking heavily, took a nap in the backyard of their home in Devon, Pennsylvania, and then shot himself through the mouth. The Vaillant children were not taken to their father's funeral. Their mother scooped up the family and moved to Arizona. They never saw their house again.

I know those childrens' feelings of grief, desolation, and abandonment. You never get over them. After a child loses a parent—especially to suicide—nothing is ever simple again. Nothing can ever be taken for granted. You might live a "normal life," but your heart is forever broken. And if your other parent is absent physically or emotionally, the trauma deepens and ramifies throughout your life.

"My former husband killed himself," Diane says. She too has been traumatized by the suicide of a man she loved.

Sorrow silently floods the room. Ancient sadness over my father's suicide wells up in my eyes, and I freeze. I don't want to share my own grief openly in this setting; I don't want to intrude—like some clichéd sports announcer—and ask how it feels to remember and share these suicides. I hope that Vaillant will walk toward me on the bridge of intimacy over the waters of grief. He doesn't.

Instead, Vaillant turns again to the intellect. "I think in a psychoanalytic way," he says, "my father's death happened when I was two." That was when Vaillant's mother left him for 3 months with a nurse who spoke only Spanish. He was, he says, "terrified of being abandoned."

While Vaillant's research and writing have championed the importance of intimacy and love, his own life has been besieged by difficulty in sustaining them. I am not the only one to see that Vaillant has been "plagued by distance and strife in his relationships," as Joshua Shenk writes in a profile of Vaillant in The Atlantic in 2009. Shenk describes him as "an optimist marinated in tragedy."

Vaillant's personality was forged on the anvil of his father's suicide by the hammer of his mother's suffering. In 1970, Vaillant divorced his first wife, with whom he had four children in 15 years. He met his second wife, with whom he had one child, at a conference in Australia. In the early 1990s, he left his second wife for a woman working on the Grant Study. Later, he returned to his second wife. Diane is his fourth wife. At one time or another, four of his five children stopped speaking to him.

Despite or because of this personal turmoil, Vaillant turned to the positive dimensions of psychiatry, psychology, and religious or spiritual experience. The titles of three of his books about growing old—Aging Well, Triumphs of Experience, and Spiritual Evolution—reflect his emphasis on positive emotions and their importance as people grow older.

Vaillant's worldview can be characterized as "spiritual but not religious," a perspective shared by as many as one-third of Americans. According to him, spirituality is "the amalgam of the positive emotions that bind us to other human beings—and to our experience of 'God' as we may understand Her/Him." He has very little interest in religious dogma or institutions, except insofar they cultivate faith, hope, and love as vehicles to the transcendent. As a scientist, Vaillant tries to demonstrate that spirituality is based in biology. The positive emotions that make up spirituality are grounded in our evolutionary heritage. They originate in the mammalian capacity for unselfish parental love.

Vaillant's personal spiritual evolution began in a family characterized by a "hodge-podge" of religious traditions. Descended from New England's Protestant elite, his parents first went to a Unitarian church, he says, because his father was "enough of an unbeliever" that no other church would have them. His mother was an Episcopalian. They sent George to the elite Congregationalist Phillips Exeter Academy, where, he says, "you had to go to church." By age 25, Vaillant decided that Unitarianism was "cheating" because it demanded "absolutely no commitment." He was baptized and confirmed in the Episcopal Church.

Vaillant says that he stopped going when it was just too much for him and his first wife to dress four children in their snow gear and get to church on time. He moved decisively toward an unchurched spirituality when he worked in a hospital research program that required him to attend Alcohol Anonymous (AA) meetings. His research led to two books on the "natural history of alcoholism." Vaillant was drawn to the spirituality of these AA meetings. Initially, he claims, he had no personal interest in the program at all (although his father's drinking probably lurked in his psyche). But he was "stunned by the recovery," he observed in the meetings over time. "You saw people in meetings that had absolutely no reason to be resilient," he tells me, "but being in AA clearly worked."

The next major turn in Vaillant's spiritual journey came when he encountered the great televangelist Robert Schuller, whose world-famous Crystal Cathedral—the largest glass building in the world—sits a few miles away from his home in Orange County. Not long after Vaillant moved to Orange to be with Diane, she was looking after her mother and trying to find day care for her 3-year-old daughter. One morning, she drove by a large complex with a "really beautiful, expensive playground" and discovered that it was part of the preschool of the Crystal Cathedral. Although she had been raised as a strict Lutheran, Diane began attending services at the Crystal Cathedral. Her initial hesitation over the "loosey-goosey theology" quickly dissolved and gave way to powerful positive feelings generated by the grandeur of the organ and the soulful power of the choir. It was not a matter of belief, she says, but of Schuller's charismatic presence and the music that swept her up into an experience of oneness with God and the universe. George followed suit.

Schuller's Crystal Cathedral opened in 1980. The building seated almost 3,000 worshipers and 1,000 singers and musicians. It also functioned as a television studio for his "Hour of Power" broadcasts, which reached more than 7.5 million viewers in the mid-1980s. Schuller's message answered a broad cultural yearning, not for salvation in the next life but for success in this life. He preached the gospel of positive thinking, self-healing, and self-improvement. His ministry was spiritual and religious at the same time.

"What I liked about Schuller's church," Diane explains,

> was that it was my first experience of hearing someone—not that I didn't believe in sin—but not just focus on sin. He turned it around and talked about the power of the gospel, the power of belief, the power of faith in terms of positive effects on the psyche, and so he was interested in positive psychology.

Positive religion appealed to George as well. It reinforced his positive approach to psychiatry and psychology. It gave him personal experience and ammunition against the traditional forms of psychiatry that focused only on pathology and illness.

"I'm looking forward to seeing the church after we finish," I say. "I'll drive down there."

"It's something," Diane says.

I am interested in how Valliant thinks about the links between spirituality, sexuality, and wisdom. So I circle back to the topic of his impotence. "I feel enormously apologetic to Diane," he says. "But the nice thing is that when people write about me now, they call me wise. At 50 when I could still screw like a bunny, nobody said I was wise." Vaillant is alluding to the traditional idea that the decline of sexual potency creates room for the growth of wisdom. But in today's hypersexualized, commercial culture, the title "wise old man" is often a dubious honor conferred on those who are no longer sexually potent or physically powerful.

In popular culture, wisdom is little more than a soft bone thrown to old dogs who have lost their teeth. In the age of Viagra, "real" men are expected to continue performing sexually, to view impotence as a medical problem. In contrast, none of the old men to whom I spoke showed any interest in using drugs to "treat" their impotence, which they view as a natural and normal occurrence.

In real life, wisdom is more than a soft bone, but no one can quite say what it is. Wisdom may be the outcome of living a good life. Or it may be a consciously pursued goal that results in a good life. Does wisdom increase with age? Perhaps, but not automatically. Scholars argue endlessly about the definition of wisdom and how to identify a wise person. "To be wise about wisdom we need to accept that wisdom does—and wisdom does not—increase with age," writes Vaillant in *Aging Well*. Like all of life's deepest questions, wisdom eludes any simple formulation. Perhaps this is why Vaillant hesitates when I press him on this topic.

"Are you a wise man?" I ask.

He pauses for a moment.

"I consider myself exactly the same as I was when I was fifteen," he says. "I've never changed. I always knew better than anybody else. But nobody else noticed I was wise until I got over 75, and my wife still doesn't even suspect it."

Vaillant is half-joking, but I take his answer seriously and tell him that his answer reminds me of the Talmudic saying that a man who is a fool in his youth is a fool when he is old, while a man who is wise when he is young is wise when he is old.

"I don't think that's how it goes, no," he says, meaning that the Talmudic view sees people as static and leaves no room for individual growth and development. Findings from the Grant Study, among others, leave no doubt that people can change and grow—although it isn't possible to predict who will grow and who will remain the same.

"But you still didn't answer my question about whether you are a wise man," I press him.

"He's very good at not answering questions," laughs Diane.

"But seriously, are you a wise man?"

I begin to realize that Vaillant is not going to answer this question. A wise man will never say he is wise. That is for others to say. Calling yourself wise violates the humility and acceptance of ambiguity and uncertainty that lie at the very core of wisdom.

Although he shies away from the label "wise," Vaillant does like to dispense the good news about aging that emerged from his research. Our culture is deeply afraid of aging. Depression stalks midlife. Vaillant wants us to know that things get better. He tells me that he hopes my book will "teach the baby boomers that cellulite is a passing disease like acne, and what's exciting about being 80 is you're less depressed than you were at 60."

For many people, the idea that "you're less depressed" at age 80 than at age 60 is not exactly a ringing endorsement of aging. It does, however, express the mix of realism and optimism that gives Vaillant's work the ring of authenticity. Once you hit age 90, he says, "you're on the clock. . . . Depression comes . . . when you're dying." But not always, Diane reminds him. There are also the fortunate men, hardy ones, who live and work right up till the end, when they fall apart "all at once and nothing first," as Oliver Wendell Holmes put it.

Vaillant's accomplishment here is not that he has solved the problems of growing old (his own or anyone else's) but that his work reduces the fear and negativity that surround aging in American culture. He sees our interview as a way of spreading the news of positive aging. "This is for your book, sir," he says to me. "The popular young person's view is that the old are lonely because they're ugly and have wrinkles. . . . Who would want to talk to them?"

More of us, he hopes. By listening and talking with old people, younger people can let go of negative stereotypes. They can become less "scared of old people and learn from them rather than wondering why they are rigid."

Vaillant includes himself among those who can learn from elders walking ahead of us on the ever-lengthening journey of life. As do I. I am talking with men like Vaillant, who are 15 or 20 years older than I am. And he, in turn, has been studying men who are 10–20 years older than he is. We are both in search of a good old age.

After I leave Vaillant's house, I drive over to the Crystal Cathedral to see the site of worship so important to George, Diane, and millions of others. Shaped like a four-pointed star with 10,000 glass panes glued to the structure's exterior, the Cathedral sits on 40 acres of land. I pull into the parking lot and shield my eyes from the glare of the setting sun, reflected off what seems like a galaxy of glass. The Cathedral is empty now, waiting to be refurbished by the Catholic Church, which bought it in 2012 after the aged Schuller was forced to declare bankruptcy due to overspending, changing styles of religious broadcasting, and the sad story of his family's failure to manage his succession. I wonder whether this financial bankruptcy signals a potential religious bankruptcy lurking in the unacknowledged shadows of positive thinking—or positive aging. For every boom there is a bust.

I drive back to my hotel, trying to understand the encounter I've had with Vaillant. I am frustrated by the discrepancy between his ideas about intimacy and my experience of him as a man I couldn't quite connect with, a brilliant scholar who uses humor or intellect to avoid descriptions of experience or expression of feelings. Like me, Vaillant has been molded by his father's suicide, his personality shaped, contorted, and constricted in adapting to its trauma. I know from experience how the heart can shut down on a dime to avoid the pain of another love lost. I have worked in therapy for years to keep my heart open. I do this very well in film interviews, oral histories, and conversations for this book. But in daily life, my heart often goes into hiding and waits for signs that it will not be broken.

I order a beer at the hotel bar. When I get back upstairs to my room, I take off my shoes and sit up against the headboard of the double bed. I am exhausted. I open my laptop and write these words about how hard it is to live up to our best selves:

> What kind of an old man is George Vaillant? I think that George Vaillant is a wise scholar who struggles to embody the wisdom he articulates. He is not the only one who struggles. We all commute between our ideals and our realities. We are confused. We shuttle back and forth between emerging understandings and ideals and the limitations of our bodies and our minds. When I ask questions of an old man, he sometimes restates an old idea or story. Sometimes he articulates a desire or a wish or a hope or a fear or a sadness. Sometimes he thinks out loud and readjusts as he goes, perhaps straying into a new thought or re-burying a long denied reality. In my best conversations with these men, we both learn something new about ourselves and about each other.

The idea is to keep learning.

CHAPTER 4 | Red Duke
*The Cowboy Surgeon*

The first time I take the elevator to the fourth floor of the medical school building for an appointment to interview Dr. Red Duke, his door is locked. I ask the Surgery Department staff across the hall where he is. Someone pages him. He is operating on a patient in the emergency room, but he will be up in a minute to apologize and reschedule. I sit on the folding table outside his office, swinging my legs and playing with my iPhone. When I look up, he is coming toward me in green scrubs and old sneakers, wearing his famous once red but now mostly white mustache. Still thin and wiry at age 85, Red Duke is hunched over a bit, and there is a hitch in his gait. He peers at me through wire-rimmed glasses, swirling his ever-present coffee around in a Styrofoam cafeteria cup. There is a drop of dried red blood on his chin.

I am excited about interviewing this larger-than-life surgeon whom some call "John Wayne in scrubs." I am also nervous: We have almost nothing in common. Duke, like all surgeons, is a man of action. I am a man of reflection. He is a Southern Baptist. I am a Northern Jew. Duke is a Texan's Texan and I am a Connecticut Yankee. Duke has an almost preternatural confidence in his own existence and his place in the world. I have never been able to take my existence for granted. He is 85. I'm 65. I don't think of myself as old, but we do have one thing in common: I too walk with a hitch in my gait. In a month, my old arthritic hip will be replaced by a new metallic one.

James Henry Duke, Jr., was born in 1928 in the tiny town of Ennis, Texas. He grew up hunting and fishing in the countryside, where his curly locks earned him the nickname Red. As a teenager, Duke became an Eagle Scout and earned money by picking cotton, digging ditches, and selling papers for the *Dallas Morning News* and *The Saturday Evening Post*. After high school in nearby Hillsboro, he went to college at Texas A&M and then served a 2-year tour of duty in Germany as a tank officer in the 2nd Armored Division of the US Army. To satisfy his father's demand, Duke enrolled in the Southwestern Baptist Theological Seminary in Fort Worth, where he graduated with a divinity degree and was ordained in 1955.

From the beginning, Red wanted to be a doctor. At age 27, he enrolled in medical school at The University of Texas Southwestern in Dallas and graduated in 1960, at age 31. After stints at Columbia University and in Jalalabad, Afghanistan, he joined the faculty of the medical school at The University of Texas at Houston in 1972, where he has lived and worked ever since. In 1976, Red founded the nation's second emergency helicopter air medical program, known as Life Flight, which has flown more than 120,000 patient missions since its inception. In April 2014, he was still Chief of the Trauma Clinic.

Duke's celebrity comes mainly from 18 years of hosting and starring in the syndicated TV series, *Dr. Red Duke's Health Reports*. But his first encounter with history took place on November 22, 1963, at Dallas's Parkland Memorial Hospital, where John F. Kennedy and Texas Governor John Connally were taken after they'd been shot. The Chief of Surgery paged "STET" to his team—a rare message of urgency—and Duke, a 35-year-old surgery resident, rushed to the emergency room.

First, Duke walked past President Kennedy, who was lying on a gurney surrounded by senior surgeons. Then he walked across the hall and turned his attention to John Connally, who was lying unattended in a separate operating room. Duke put a tube in Connally's chest and readied him for the surgery that saved his life. Historian Douglas Brinkley interpreted the situation this way:

> Red Duke is a trauma doctor. Well, he was there when our nation went into trauma. When you think about what the doctors dealt with that day at Parkland, you know, they did a great job because Red Duke recognized "Kennedy's dead, I gotta go work on John Connally," who not only went on to survive, but also to have decades active in American politics.

Duke and Connally went on to become close friends and lifelong hunting partners.

Still, Duke is not fully at peace with what happened. One image still haunts him: the red roses that Jackie Kennedy had been carrying earlier that day. "As I walked out of the room," he recalled in a CBS Evening News interview, "I pulled my gloves off and threw 'em into a kick basin, and those roses were upside down in that kick basin, and my gloves fell over it."

When you walk into Red Duke's office, the first thing you notice is the absence of wall space. There are pictures of great mountain ranges and cowboys, gag photos, honorific plaques, and many pictures of Duke—on horseback with his auburn red hair and beard; as a great frontiersman modeled after Davy Crockett; on a snow sled pulled by Alaskan huskies; carrying slain caribou, mountain sheep, and deer. And there are mounted trophies, mostly of mountain sheep with huge curled horns and deer with many-pointed antlers. I want to know more about the place of hunting in his life and how it changed as he's gotten older. I ask Duke if he would still hunt today.

"Oh, yeah."

"What would you hunt? Where would you go?"

"Well, I'd probably just go deer hunting. I don't really care about killing anything. I just want to get out in the brush."

When he himself was a young buck, Duke's favorite outings were to hunt wild sheep in the mountains—hunting for the big heads that are mounted on his office walls. Duke emphasizes the mountain scenery and the challenge of bagging "a big one because it's hard to find them. And the attraction of the mountains is, I think, the mountains."

Duke grew up hunting and killing animals. For him, hunting is not violence but a form of sport, a means of obtaining food, or a form of conservation. His father first took him hunting at the age of 7: "He'd use me as a bird dog. I always said he was too cheap to buy a dog because he had me, and now he could point me out there. And besides that, I could clean and cook the birds, too." When Duke was a child in rural Texas, no one thought twice about killing animals. During World War II, his family raised chickens. "And every Sunday after church I went out and got a pullet, wrung her neck, scalded it, picked it, gutted it, and gave it to Mother to cook, and I didn't think anything about it." Today, Duke is virtually a vegetarian. He's not uncomfortable with hunting, but it doesn't attract his interest either. "I don't give a shit about killing anything," he says,

I'm a frustrated artist, and I really want to get out there and paint. I've painted off and on—mainly off—all my life. As I've grown older and had a little better understanding about the world and life, I've become more and more conscious of the actual awesomeness or miracle of life itself in any form.

Duke has adapted to his body's changes by making a few concessions:

I do like to go out into West Texas and go hunting, but I haven't been able to. I don't do any long operations anymore because my back has kind of gotten bad. I had a laminectomy several years ago, and in the meantime something's twisted up back there. My right paraspinous muscle has hypertrophied just from trying to hold it up, and I can't lean over for a long time.

"Anything else about being old that's different than being younger?" I ask. His answer speaks volumes about the meaning of manhood to him:

Well, yeah. Hell, things hurt. God Almighty. My back hurts, my shoulder hurts. I've got an iron shoulder in here. I slipped on a glacier in Alaska one time and got it operated on. It was really crazy. I love being in the mountains up there . . . that's a great place, man. I don't know why I didn't go to live there because their idea is—their motto is, "Why not?" Don't ever bring it up if you aren't willing to do it or else back down. They're just a tougher bunch than what you've got around here.

Set among the trophies, pictures, plaques, and outdoor scenes are pictures of key mentors—Dr. Truman Blocker, a powerful army surgeon who became president of the University of Texas Medical Branch; Dr. Donald Seldin, an internist trained at Yale University and an intellectual father of the University of The Texas Southwestern Medical Center; and Dr. Robert Shaw, the thoracic surgeon who oversaw Governor Connelly's surgery during the Kennedy assassination.

The walls in Duke's dark office reflect a long and crowded life, with little room for anything but his all-consuming medical work, his patients, his hunting and outdoor life—and these days his multicolored Catahoula dog named Jake. The walls also suggest a crowding out of personal space, of intimacy. Married and divorced twice, he has little time or interest in romantic relationships. "I like women," he says,

but I wouldn't want to mess with one every day. Most of the women you encounter here—in this world, in this town—have been raised in the city, and their values are kind of messed up. I think they're pretty superficial. They're more materialistic.

Duke has been living in the hospital for 20 years, ever since he received death threats in 1994. "I was right here, sitting at this desk, and a lawyer called me," he says. The lawyer was interviewing the family of a man who had been removed from life support. The man was a cocaine-abusing alcoholic, according to Duke, and had been sick for a long time. "We got him over all of it, but by the end he didn't have anything left in here"—Duke points to his head—"no lights on, nobody home." Fortunately for Duke, the man's wife and sister were both nurses in Houston—at MD Anderson and Ben Taub—and they understood that the man was brain dead. They decided to remove the man's life support.

Although the rest of his family understood that there were no grounds for a lawsuit, the patient's brother began talking about suing and "killing Dr. Duke." Duke called the chief of police and the sheriff. For the next 3 months, "I had a cop living with me every day and had dinner with one every night. I thought it was kinda stupid for me to go in my little apartment out there," Duke says, "so I started sleeping in my office, and I got to where I liked it." He moved to a call room and has lived there ever since. Ten years later, Duke's daughter brought him a puppy he named Jake. Jake, whose muzzle is turning white, is his closest companion. Duke smiles and says, "He's better behaved than any kid I've ever had."

Duke gets up at 4:30 a.m. every day and takes Jake to doggy day care. Then he goes to the physician's dining hall for breakfast and takes his Styrofoam cup of black coffee to morning report on the hospital Trauma Service. Except for a short lunch in the physicians' dining room at Memorial Hermann Hospital, the rest of Duke's day is filled with surgery, teaching, and meetings. After work, he'll go out to a local restaurant. Although he still enjoys Texas barbecued ribs once in a while, he is careful these days to eat "fruits, vegetables, a lot of fish, and a little bit of chicken."

After dinner, Duke returns to the hospital to read and respond to mail—mostly snail mail; Duke remains a stranger to the digital world. When his patients are moved from the emergency room to a hospital floor, he visits with every one of them, and he writes notes in their charts. The electronic medical record, he thinks, is more about making money than ensuring good medical care. "I'm one of these old docs that believes that you ought to follow the patients," he tells me,

> I don't leave town because I see them every day, seven days a week, and I write a long note. And now I think it's basically driven by greed because these electronic records have got all these boxes you have to check, and you are supposed to scribble something down here and there. I don't know how they get away with charging for it. I wouldn't pay anybody to do that because you can't figure out your patient—you can read those all day long and not know what's going on.

Duke takes a similar interest in the real lives of his students and residents (those newly minted doctors still in training). As a professor and clinical teacher, his style differs little from the intimidating, demanding way that he himself was trained as a surgeon. Former trainees describe him as a terrifying taskmaster who rarely cracked a smile and berated students for not knowing answers or for making mistakes. Duke believes that "anybody can understand almost anything, no matter how technical, if the language used by the communicator is such that the person is familiar with it." For more than 18 years, he put these words into practice in front of a national audience, first on an Emmy Award Winning episode of NBC's *Lifeline*, then on PBS's program *Bodywatch*, and finally (and most prominently) on *Dr. Red Duke's Health Reports*, which was produced by The University of Texas and distributed nationally.

In a 1982 segment, for instance, Duke can be seen explaining hyperthyroidism by way of auto care. Looking up from the hood of a blue car, Duke steps away from a circle of mechanics and faces the camera:

> Everybody knows that if you race your car engine too much for too long something is gonna wear out and the same thing is true of your body. If some condition causes your body engine to burn its fuel too fast, something'll break. One cause for problems like weight loss or rapid heartbeat is an overactive thyroid.

In a segment from 1991, he uses a jackhammer to illustrate how kidney stones are treated. Wearing thick boots, gloves, and a hardhat as he hammers away on a patch of concrete, Duke stops, takes off his hard hat, and looks up: "Now, you probably wonder: What's he doing messing with a jackhammer? A jackhammer works by vibrating and cutting apart the ground. It's like doctors vibrating and breaking down kidney stones in the human body."

Duke was not only interested in explaining the technical aspects of medicine in laymen's terms in these spots. In one segment, "Time Away," Duke holds a cup of coffee in front of a fence on which two cowboys sit:

> How often do you come to the end of a wild hectic day, having dealt with jillions of details, trying to be responsible, and then you can't remember what, if anything, you've accomplished? This goes on for days and weeks and months. And then you realize that, throughout all of this, you haven't devoted any time to yourself, your loved ones, or your friends.

In another segment, "Burn Out," Duke sits on a stump by a campfire with his cowboy hat on his knee:

Most of us live and work in what some folks have called an unnatural and unhealthy concrete jungle. We're constantly bombarded by streams of information, regulation, traffic, and just general problems with our society. It's little wonder that some of us burn out. We need a rest from it.

In both segments, Duke delivers his message with such heartful surety that you are compelled to believe the cowboy doctor when he strolls along a handmade fence and says,

You know, there's something really calming about the end of the day in the woods. There's a brook running around over here behind me. There's night creatures just beginning their chorus. It's the sort of thing that really does calm down your soul. It's the sort of thing I hope you can find a little bit of tonight.

There are other times, however, when Duke appears as a very different sort of cowboy. In one 1989 video, the door to the trauma wing swings open to allow a grave, white-coated Duke to walk in and stare directly at the camera: "This country's unrecognized trauma epidemic is shameful. Trauma destroys more potential years of life than cancer, heart disease, and infection put together. And the emotional and economic costs are staggering." In another, from the same year, he stands in an empty hallway of a hospital with his elbow on a counter as if he were in a saloon: "It's hard to believe, but between 30 and 70% of the people that die in hospitals after a car wreck die unnecessarily. Why? Because they're not taken to a hospital that really takes care of them properly soon enough." Then, in what seems almost like a sales pitch, he explains how regionalized trauma systems work and why we need to develop them in order to provide care for people in urban and rural areas. Granted, an effective system is expensive. But the highest risk groups for trauma are children and young adults. "The child saved from a needless death on some back road just might be yours," he says, as a dreadful auto wreck appears on the screen. Then, he appears one more time in front of an ambulance, wearing a suit and tie and holding a single flower as he looks unflinchingly into the camera as the wind whips through his hair. "The symbol of the American Trauma Society is the broken flower because that's just exactly what trauma does," he says, snapping the stem in two. "It breaks and kills our kids just when they're about to bloom."

Watching these videos in succession, you might get the impression that Duke has become a caricature of himself—the cowboy surgeon who always rides to the rescue or who needs to be home on the range. But Red is the real thing. He exemplifies the gerontologist's truism that as we get older, we become more like ourselves. And as I came to realize, he lives rather than speaks the answers to questions about what it means to be an old man. The "answer" is the story of his life.

If medical students today don't always appreciate his style, they universally respect Red Duke. Caring for trauma patients requires immediate decision-making with little room for error. Duke is nothing if not decisive. The Life Flight program, which he founded in 1976, completes 3,000 missions per year and is one of the busiest in the country. Every day, big red whirling helicopters fly patients onto the Memorial Hermann Hospital roof. They are brought down to the trauma bay, where three stretchers separated by curtains are ready and waiting. When a patient arrives, Duke stands silently at the edge of the bed, waiting to see how the senior resident starts the trauma protocol. Then he starts barking commands, explaining procedures, and demanding actions from the entire team. Although he still runs the Trauma Clinic, Duke doesn't take night calls anymore:

> I used to get by fine with 3 or 4 hours of sleep. I can't do that anymore. My battery runs down quicker, and it doesn't charge as fast. So I have to sleep more than I used to, and I may take a nap in the day, too. But I frequently just keep going.

Duke's presence pervades the place even when he is not there. Beneath the foot of each trauma bed, a pair of cowboy bootprints is etched into the cement floor. They are painted in red.

Red Duke has spent a lifetime practicing and demonstrating the tough, decisive action and knowledge of a trauma surgeon. His job is to stabilize patients brought by ambulance or helicopter into the emergency room and whose lives are threatened by the results of violence or accidents—gunshot wounds, stab wounds, blunt trauma to the head, car accidents, explosions, warfare, burns, and drug overdose or other forms of toxicity. Trauma surgeons lead teams of nurses and other support staff. They must act quickly and often with inadequate knowledge to resuscitate, stabilize, evaluate, and transfer patients to the intensive care unit and eventually hospital rooms for appropriate care. Duke is one of a disappearing breed—a trauma surgeon who actually follows and cares for his patients once they are moved onto a regular hospital floor.

It is drawing close to the end of my scheduled interview with him. Every day at 2 p.m., Duke goes to the physician's dining room at Memorial Hermann, gathers up the leftover food from lunch, and takes it to a nursing station in the hospital. At 5 minutes before 2 p.m., he excuses himself and walks over to the hospital to deliver food to the nurses. From there, he'll round on his next hospitalized patient and then the next and the next until he goes to pick up Jake at doggy day care, comes back to the hospital to sleep, and does it all again tomorrow.

Dr. Red Duke died on August 25, 2015. He was buried alongside other luminaries in the Texas State Cemetery. At the bottom of his tombstone are inscribed the words of a salty old Texan:

*Piss on the fire, call in the dogs. This hunt is over.*

| Sherwin Nuland

*The Old Man Who Was Young and Strong*

One September afternoon in his 71st year, Dr. Sherwin Nuland was riding a crowded New York subway with his wife Sally and his daughter Molly when a young man groped for Molly's bottom. Nuland backed into the man and pushed him up against the subway door. Then he felt a hand surreptitiously sliding down the right-hand pocket of his khaki pants, searching for money. Nuland shoved his own hand down around the man's hand, squeezed as hard as he could, and felt the sickening sensation of bones cracking. The man shrieked in pain and ran out the subway door at the next stop.

This incident opens Nuland's book, *The Art of Aging*, published when he was age 76. It reveals a deep concern about virility and strength, something still on his mind when we spoke 5 years later in his rambling colonial house just outside New Haven, Connecticut.

I grew up in New Haven, where Nuland practiced surgery and taught at Yale University for many years. After two decades of work as a surgeon, he gave up medical practice, turned to full-time writing, and became an internationally celebrated author. Nuland was a friend of friends, so I knew him as "Shep." I got to know him better when I invited him to speak at the Institute for Medical Humanities in Galveston, Texas, where I was working in the 1990s. Of Nuland's many books, I especially admired the award-winning *How We Die*—a classic meditation on death and dying. Nuland wrote on topics ranging from the history of medicine to Leonardo Da Vinci, Moses Maimonides, and his own powerful memoir *Lost in America*. He thought *The Art of Aging* was his best book.

It is mid-afternoon when I arrive at New York City's LaGuardia Airport and rent a car to drive to New Haven and meet with Shep. He and his wife

Sally have invited me for dinner and to spend the night. I really have no idea where this book project is going. Shep is only my third interview. To make things worse, I lost his phone number and the directions to his house and have no idea where *I* am going. I fume inside the airport's Enterprise Rent-A-Car lot and wonder what to do next. It is getting foggy and dark, and rush-hour traffic from New York is already clogging Interstate 95 northbound to Connecticut. Finally, I call my old friend Steve Stein, who gives me Shep's number and directions to his house. I call and tell Shep that I'll be late.

When I pull in front of his house 3 hours later, it is dark and snowing lightly. I wheel my suitcase to his front door. Shep—a tall, still well-built and handsome man at age 81—welcomes me, puts the suitcase at the foot of the stairs, and ushers me into the kitchen. There he and Sally, who is about 20 years his junior, serve me homemade chicken soup, salad, and bread. As we begin talking, I turn on my recorder. Shep sits on my left. Sally sits across the table opposite from me.

From the start, Nuland resists the idea that he is an old man. "I just don't see myself as old," he says. He has recently finished reading 83-year-old Donald Hall's article "Out the Window," in *The New Yorker*. And he is rattled. Hall—America's poet laureate in 2006–2007—grew up around the corner from Shep's house and walked to nearby Spring Glen Elementary School as a child. Now he is wheelchair bound and writing sardonically about being patronized or treated as if he were invisible. "When we turn eighty," says Hall,

we understand that we are extraterrestrial. If we forget for a moment that we are old, we are reminded when we try to stand up, or when we encounter someone young. . . . People's response to our separateness can be callous, can be good-hearted, and is always condescending.

A pained look comes over Nuland's face. "To think that this guy is within 2 years of my age and his physical life is over." He thinks to himself out loud: "Gee, I'm in terrific shape. I can do anything, but my God, maybe in 2 years, I'll be like that."

In fact, 2 years later, Nuland would die a painful death from prostate cancer, and Donald Hall would still be alive in his wheelchair.

"That piece made me look outside of myself and try to see what people who don't know me see," Nuland continues,

Like, I go to the gym, and what does the 23-year-old girl on the next machine think of what I am? She doesn't see the guy I see. She sees an old guy with gray hair: *Isn't it nice he's trying to stay in shape?* I see the same young, vibrant guy

I was in my 20s or 30s working really hard to keep my muscles in shape, to make more muscle. In other words, what's inside me is ongoing progress and growth. What goes on inside of her when she sees me is a gray-haired guy over the hump who is trying to stay alive.

Nuland's view of himself as young and vibrant presents an important counterstory that resists the view of ourselves as falling apart, going downhill, ready to fall into the grave. This counterstory may be true, but it is only a partial truth. If we think it is the whole truth, we deny a piece of our own reality. We become partial strangers to ourselves, as Sigmund Freud relates in an anecdote about traveling on an overnight train in his early 60s. When Freud closed the door to his sleeping compartment, he was startled by the image of a strange old man staring at him. It was his own reflection in the mirror.

As we grow older, we all harbor a suppressed shadow self that can catch us off guard when we glance in the mirror and don't recognize ourselves, or when we are driving at night and can't quite see, or when we fall stepping off a curb—or worse, when we lose a partner, have a stroke or a heart attack, or receive a diagnosis of cancer. I ask Shep about such fears catching up with him. "Those thoughts really cross my mind very rarely," he says.

Like Shep Nuland, we all need to resist internalizing our culture's pervasive fear and hatred of growing old. But we also need to acknowledge our fear and recover the shadow side of ourselves. Not because the fears and shadows are more true than the positive stories we tell about ourselves. But because they are real. And because we cannot become whole if we are ashamed and deny or hide these pieces of ourselves rather than acknowledge and share them in relationships of love and care.

As I sit at my dining room table writing this chapter, a few years after my conversation with Shep, I live these issues every day. Two weeks ago, my orthopedic surgeon, Dr. Gregory Stocks, slit open the muscles holding the top of my right leg bone to my pelvic bone and pulled them apart. He sawed off the head of my femur and hammered in a metal shaft topped by a shiny new ball. Then he scraped out what was left of the cartilage in the socket, glued in a plastic one, and popped the metal ball back into the new socket. He sewed up the muscles and skin and made me a new right hip. The anesthesia team kept me in the recovery room for 2 hours, searching for the right pain medication to keep down my angry cursing and shouting. Or so I am told.

This surgery is the latest in a 3-year siege of health problems: surgery to replace my other hip, a 6-month bout of mycoplasma pneumonia, followed by a relapse and another surgery to relieve chronic back pain from severe osteoarthritis.

These are problems that Shep Nuland, at age 81, has been able to keep at bay. In my late 60s, they plague me. What happened to my identity as a strong, youthful man? With good medical care and hard work in physical therapy, I am determined to return to my usual strength and endurance. But perhaps I will become wheelchair bound. As I return to work and spend more time out in public, I feel good. I portray an image of confidence, optimism, and good cheer. At the same time, at home and with friends, I share, from time to time, the truth of my physical pain, anxiety, and sense of loss that come with having a body no longer young.

It is difficult to find the right balance between darkness and light—acknowledging the negative and accentuating the positive. I do not control the outcome of these painful attacks on the strength and integrity of my hips and legs. But I have to work physically and spiritually as if I do and accept whatever comes next. And I need to stay focused on the well-being of others.

The core of my conversation with Shep revolved not around being an old man (since he didn't see himself as old) but around *becoming* a man—an American man. Nuland was born Shepsel Ber Nudelman into a poor, Jewish, immigrant family in 1930. Yiddish was the spoken language of the household, which consisted of Shep, his parents, his brother, his aunt, and his grandmother. All six of them lived in a four-room flat at 1215 Olmstead Avenue in a quiet neighborhood of the Bronx that was later bulldozed to make way for the Cross Bronx Expressway. Shep learned English from Irish Catholic nuns in New York public schools. It was a "huge transformation," he wrote in his memoir, "because it was the opening to the New World." And like many upwardly mobile immigrants or children of immigrants, he changed his name.

Shepsel Ber Nudelman changed his name to Sherwin Nuland in 1946— long before our era of multiple identities, when it is commonplace to be considered an African American, a Jewish American, an Asian American, a Muslim American, and so on. For Shep, becoming a man meant becoming an *American* man—an intensely competitive process of upward assimilation and entry into the circles of elite white Protestant men. After undergraduate school at New York University, Nuland moved to New Haven to become a medical student at Yale, where he did his surgery residency and became chief resident—the highest possible accomplishment at one of the most prestigious universities in the world. By his 30s, Nuland was a successful American man by any measure.

When I ask him about the meaning of manhood, Nuland speaks like a surgeon:

A man is decisive. A man studies all the facts very quickly, analyzes them, comes to a decision and acts on it. It's not enough to think. You've got to act. That's part of it. I've always been impressed when I read something in which the author somehow makes the distinction between thinking about a problem and acting on it because I've always felt that action is what really counts.

But underneath Shep's self-confidence lies a terrible vulnerability.

"Who taught you what it is to be a man?"

He glares at me. "Nobody. Nobody, nobody, nobody. Absolutely nobody. That was the goddamn trouble!"

Shep spent much of his life trying to overcome the shame of his father's failure, fear of his own, and the deeply internalized stigma of being Jewish and poor. His mother died when he was 11 years old. His father Meyer Nudelman couldn't read or write English, so Shep had to complete all kinds of official documents and correspondence for him. For many years, he also attended dutifully to his father's health problems, especially Meyer's growing inability to control his limbs due to neurological deterioration that Shep later discovered was a result of syphilis. Worse, his father Meyer was a terrible bully who flew into unpredictable rages that terrified Shep and left him with dark, lifelong fears and vulnerability to major depression.

In his early 40s, Nuland spent 2 years in a mental hospital in Hartford, Connecticut, during which time his physicians seriously considered a lobotomy before giving him round after round of electroshock therapy. Miraculously and with much help from a psychotherapist, he recovered from this disabling depression and a failed marriage and rebuilt his life as a surgeon in New Haven.

As a young man, Shep says, he developed an arrogant, condescending, and brittle persona—a mask that covered the inferiority he felt for being a "Jew boy" and the terrors of a little boy still helpless against his father's rages.

Shep was also brought up as a bigot. "In my household," he says, "blacks were called *schwartza* [the equivalent of "nigger"] and every Christian was a *goy* [a gentile] . . . and a *goy* by definition was stupid. . . . *Goyim* (plural) were murderers. You had to worry about them all the time, and this was inculcated in me by my grandmother."

Nuland's family was among the 2 million Jews who emigrated from Europe to the United States between the 1880s and World War I, drawn by opportunities or fleeing from vicious forms of anti-Semitism. Many had lived in the actual, physical form of a ghetto—an impoverished and closely regulated Jewish quarter of a Central or Eastern European city, literally surrounded by walls that set them apart from the larger Christian population. Jews in these ghettos and in rural settings were often attacked in organized massacres known as pogroms.

One day in the late 1940s, Meyer Nudelman came home from his work stitching clothes in the Ladies Garment District in Manhattan. He was clutching a copy of the Yiddish language *Jewish Daily Forward*, which was then publishing new information coming from Eastern Europe about the fate of Jews during the Holocaust. Nudelman, who had never before spoken about his family, collapsed in cries of anguish and locked himself in his bedroom. The Nazis had herded all the Jews of his hometown of Novoselitza into their small wooden homes in the Jewish quarter. They drove their armored cars around and around, firing machine guns and rockets into every home until no sound was heard. Then they burned the entire area to the ground. Not a single Jew survived.

As the evening wears on, Shep and Sally encourage me to have some dessert, and Sally refreshes my cup of tea. The conversation flows easily. But as we begin talking about Joseph Epstein's nasty review of *The Art of Aging* in *The New York Times*, they both become agitated. It is the most intense and uncomfortable moment of the night.

Epstein's review coincided with the book launch and appeared in *The New York Times* on the first Sunday in March 2007. An author can't ask for a better spot than the *Times'* Sunday Book Review section, which is also published separately and circulated a few days early. A friend of Shep's read Epstein's review ahead of time and called to warn him to soften the blow. It didn't help.

Epstein laced into Shep with the harshest personal attack I've ever seen in a book review. "The unflinchingly lucid man who wrote *Lost in America* and *How We Die* puts in only a part-time appearance in Nuland's new book," wrote Epstein,

> *The Art of Aging* feels as if it has been written by two different people: one a nononsense medical scientist and the other a Polonius-like figure who delivers a series of sermonettes in the psychobabble of the day and whom, as I read, I preferred to think of as Nudelman.

*The Art of Aging* is an advice book and consists mostly of stories and interviews with men and women who exemplify a well-lived life. I wrote a lukewarm review of it for the *Houston Chronicle*. Mercifully, I don't think he ever read it. The longest chapter, "How We Age: Body and Mind," argues that aging is not a disease but, rather, a normal physiological process of increasing vulnerability to disease, frailty, and death. Nuland does battle—correctly, I believe—with the anti-aging scientists, clinicians, drug companies, and charlatans who argue that aging is a disease that can and should be fought and conquered. He emphasizes the importance of developing one's physical strength and vitality in order to fight off biological threats and offers advice about cultivating the virtues of "wisdom, equanimity, and caring." It is up to each of us, Shep argues, to prepare for our own aging morally and spiritually as well as physically. Yet preparation is no guarantee of success.

The Epstein review ripped the Band-Aid off lingering psychic wounds from Shep's childhood:

> Everything I had built over the years just came crumbling down. I went into a profound depression, to the point where I would go up in my bed with the covers over my head. I wouldn't come down. I wouldn't leave the house. And I ended up with two brief hospitalizations, of about ten days or so and once again, electroshock therapy.

It took Shep more than 2 years to recover from the depression provoked by Epstein's review. He withdrew into his own private hell. Sally and Shep basically lived parallel lives. Somehow, Sally found the love and support and stamina to maintain her own life. "I waited for him to come back with faith that he would," she says. During that awful period, Nuland worked intensively with a psychotherapist in New Haven. When he gradually regained his bearings and mental health, Shep had finally earned the kind of wisdom he advocates in *The Art of Aging*.

I drink my tea slowly, buying time to absorb and honor his suffering before I move onto my next question.

"What is your biggest regret?" I ask.

"That I matured so late," he says instantly,

> I was really narcissistic all my life. I was a good-looking kid. I was a smart kid. I was the apple of my grandmother's and my aunt's eye. I was the favorite boy. I had a sense of self-assurance that was far beyond what I should have had growing up. I didn't allow any weaknesses in myself. I thought I was a superior human being. I was a manly man. I was the kind of man any woman would want to marry. I was the guy during residency who used to screw all the nurses.

Nuland laments that it took him so long to come to a place of genuine kindness and compassion—to grow up, as he puts it. It saddens him to think that now, just when he is learning how to live, he has so little time left.

"Earlier in my life," Shep says, "I was kind—but only to my family, my friends, and my patients." Once he achieved fame and accepted his vulnerability, he enjoyed a peace he had never experienced before. In his 70s, Shep came across Philo of Alexandria's admonition: "Be kind, because everyone you meet is fighting a great battle."

It is late. Sally has cleared the dishes. I don't want to miss my last chance.

"What should I have asked you that we didn't discuss?" I ask. "What do you want to say about being a man who is old?"

"That I'm not old," he says once more,

I'm chronologically old, but I don't think in those terms at all. I think I'm not grown up enough. . . . In no way, shape, or form do I think of myself as old—I can't. I try to. I really try to, but I can't do it. I was in the gym on Sunday morning, and I was on the cross-trainer. And from behind me, I hear a woman's voice say, "Look at those terrific legs." And I turn around. It was one of Sarah's friends who was on her way to an exercise class. . . . You know what went through my mind? Of course I have beautiful legs. I've always had beautiful legs.

When I was 13 years old, my great-aunt Marion handed me an envelope containing a letter printed in both Yiddish and English. It was dated 5 Adar Sheni (March), 1881.

"You should always be proud of your family," she said.

Aunt Marion and Uncle Sidney lived up the hill from us on Birch Drive in New Haven, Connecticut. Their two-story house always seemed dark inside. It was fiercely defended by a black spaniel named Heidi. In their garage, Marion and Sidney kept a large painted wooden circus horse, probably taken from a carousel at the Savin Rock amusement park about half an hour away. That horse was a source of endless delight even though my brother, sister, and I were rarely allowed to climb on it.

I glanced at the letter Marion gave me and put it in a desk drawer. Somehow it survived, becoming more faded by the year, inside cardboard boxes that I stuffed in closets and attics and carried with me during decades of peregrinations that took me to Rochester, Omaha, Galveston, and finally to Houston.

One hot day some 30 years later, in the summer of 1992, I came across that letter while moving from one house to another in Houston. I sat on a cardboard box and started reading. The letter was written by Elijah Joseph Solomon, a distant ancestor on my mother's side who lived in Staropole, a tiny village in what is today southern Poland. Elijah was responding to his son Symcha Trytel, who asked about their family's history. It begins:

To My Dearly Beloved Son,
First, I desire to inform you that we are all in good health, and hope to hear from you continued reports of good health and prosperity. In the

second place, I desire to let you know that I received your letter and rejoiced to read of your well-being. I also received the ten rubles for which you sent a draft. For your kindheartedness and constant remembrance of us, I thank you. . . .

What the purpose of your request is, I do not know, but it will give me great pleasure to comply with it. The account which follows below I heard from my parents of blessed memory . . . and I dare say they took just pride in relating it.

In Elijah's letter, I read stories of great rabbis, authors, scholars, and merchants—even a rabbi who put peas in his shoes at night to keep himself awake while studying Torah. I was moved by the love and pride and accomplishment and dignity of ancestors who lived and toiled in tiny little Eastern European villages hundreds of years ago.

It was a hot, sweaty day, and I had many more boxes to move and unpack. I started to fold the letter and stuff it back into its envelope when the next paragraph caught my eye. It described an event that took place in the 17th century in the Prussian village of Werbelow, where an order was given to execute all Jews in the village for using the blood of Christian babies in their Passover services. Elijah wrote,

But Rabbi Menachim Man decided to save the community at the price of his own life. He went to the authorities and solemnly declared that no one in the entire village had any guilt but he. Thus he sacrificed his life. He was named "Menachim Man the Martyr."

Menachim Man was my ancestor. He was executed for the "blood libel," an excuse used for centuries to murder thousands of Jews in Christian Europe by claiming that they used the blood of Christian babies for making matzah in the Passover ceremonies.

Sitting in my overheated attic, I read the paragraph again to make sure I understood it: My ancestor had sacrificed his life so that the Jews of the village could live. Then it hit me: I am descended from Menachim Man's children and from his children's children on down through 11 generations. If he had not sacrificed his life, I would never have been born. I would never have been conceived, drawn breath, lived, loved, and had children of my own. Nor would any of the thousands of Menachim Man's descendants.

That day in the attic, something invaded my sweaty body: I shuddered. I shook my head from side to side as if trying to rid myself of an unfathomable revelation. I fell into what Rabbi Abraham Heschel calls "radical amazement"—dread and astonishment and incredible joy that I was even alive at all. Scientists estimate that the odds of any of us ever being born are 1 in 4 trillion. This truth was no longer abstract to me. It now lived in my body and in my soul.

People have pointed out to me that this story may be apocryphal. Perhaps. But if it was not my ancestor Menachim Man, then it was someone else's Jewish ancestor who sacrificed himself.

I have decided to live as if the story is true. This means I am constantly alert to the murderous possibilities of all prejudice. It means I remind myself over and over again that life is an exceedingly rare and brief opportunity. It means that every moment is truly a gift, a passing instant of grace, a chance to work for justice, a sliver of light to keep "the soul's door open," as Emily Dickinson put it.

In 1995, my mother turned 70, I turned 46, and my daughter Emma turned 9. I began looking for a way to reprint this letter and pass the story on. My friend, the psychiatrist and printmaker Eric Avery, offered to teach me how to produce handmade paper and print and bind the letter into a little hand-sewn book. Emma came with me to make the book in Eric's Galveston studio. We cut out Hebrew and English words and phrases from my grandfather's bible, stirred them into a mix of water and cotton pulp, and rolled out sheets to dry. The words sanctified the paper. A week later, we came back and hand printed 30 copies of the letter. We sewed the pages together with a cover that my sister Patty designed.

At my mother's 80th birthday celebration, I gave the book to her, to my son Jake, and to my siblings and their children and later to my cousins and other extended family members. I fulfilled an obligation: Remember and tell your children. My great-aunt had given the story to me. Now I had given it to Emma, who helped me reproduce and pass it on to future generations.

I suspect that this family letter will sit and gather dust in many drawers until someone finds and reads it and passes it on again.

PART II | Do I Still Matter?

## CHAPTER 6

The Moral World of Paul Volcker

"This is not the kind of thing you talk about every day," I say.

"This is the kind of thing I *think* about every day."

So begins my conversation with 85-year-old Paul Volcker, the man who served as Chairman of the Federal Reserve under Presidents Carter and Reagan and later as Chairman of President Obama's Economic Recovery Advisory Board. Volcker sits behind a large granite desk in his office at the historic Rockefeller Center in Manhattan, his 6-foot, 8-inch frame genially slumped against the back of his chair. Thirty-five years ago, when the conservative and immovable Volcker took highly controversial measures to bring down soaring inflation, he was the most powerful financial official in the world. Now he's rereading my book prospectus.

I came to interview Volcker by a strange route. Two years earlier, my friend, Columbia historian Casey Blake, introduced me to Volcker's niece, who loved the project and forwarded my materials and letter requesting an interview. I never heard from him.

The next April, after a Sunday service at Riverside Church in Manhattan, my wife Thelma Jean and I were eating lunch at an Italian restaurant, one of those neat little New York City places slightly submerged below street level. Halfway through lunch, I spotted Paul Volcker sitting at a corner table with his wife Anke Dening and another couple.

"Go get him," said Thelma Jean when Volcker and his party got up to leave.

"I can't do that."

"What have you got to lose?" she said. "And besides, he's not going to turn you down. With a face like yours, no one could turn you down."

I followed Volcker's party outside, looked up at him and said, "Mr. Volcker, you won't remember me, but last year I sent a letter requesting an interview for a book I'm writing on men's experience of old age. Would you consider doing it?"

"She's the boss," he said to me pointing to Anke. "Ask her."

I gave her my name and affiliation, and she gave me her phone number and email address.

"We're traveling quite a bit in the next month or two," she said. "Send me the materials and call in July."

Now as we sit in his New York City office, I want Volcker to discuss those "things" he thinks about every day but rarely discusses: love and work life, sexuality, hopes and fears, high and low points, and regrets.

"Who do you love?" I ask.

"Who do I love? Well, I guess I'm supposed to say my wife," he says, signaling that it's not something he wants to discuss. I cannot bring myself to press the former Chairman of the Federal Reserve to tell me more about loving his wife. In any case, it would be a complicated story because his first wife died after an illness of many years and his current wife Anke was previously his assistant. So I quickly move on.

"*What* do you love?" I ask.

What do I love? I don't know. I love being involved in things because I can see old men not so involved in anything—you don't have the same incentive, the same discipline—and from one point of view that's fine, and some people want to go Florida and play golf. I'm not a golfer so I don't want to play golf, and even if I played golf I wouldn't want to get absorbed in it. I'm too old to get that absorbed in fishing, which used to be my preoccupation. But you want to feel needed—that's what you want to feel, *needed*.

Volcker doesn't feel needed when he is merely asked to lend his name or to attend a social function. "People come around, we need you for this, that and the other thing—a charity or whatever, sign this petition or whatever, or come to this meeting—and from that standpoint a lot of people come around," he says. He is used to being honored at big dinners where some foundation will sell expensive tables and bring in inspirational speakers to raise money for its cause. "But feeling needed because you're making a difference to something that's important is a little different story."

"The Volcker Rule is a pretty important thing," I say. He nods. "That's the last thing that I got involved with, because I was already somewhat involved in financial reform and at that point I had access to the President. Then I could get engaged and I was in charge."

The Volcker Rule, passed by Congress in 2010, limits US banks' ability to make certain kinds of speculative investments that are known, on Wall Street, as proprietary trading. When more than 5,000 banks failed during the Great Depression, the federal government established the Federal Deposit Insurance Corporation, which insured customers' money, and Congress passed the Glass–Steagall Act of 1933, which prohibited banks from selling stocks. When that act was repealed in 1999, Wall Street firms could once again speculate on potentially volatile products such as mortgage-backed securities and credit-default swaps.

In 2008, when these risky ventures failed and the markets crashed, the US economy plunged into its deepest recession since the 1930s. Millions lost their jobs. Huge banks, considered "too big to fail," were bailed out at taxpayers' expense. Yet within a year, senior employees at huge investment firms were again making huge salaries and receiving big bonuses—more than $16 billion at Goldman Sachs alone. The public was outraged, but Treasury Secretary Lawrence Summers refused to consider taxing profits and bonuses.

Volcker's moral sensibility first took shape in the quiet suburban town of Teaneck, New Jersey, where as a boy he looked through his kitchen window at the Empire State Building across the Hudson River. Volcker's grandparents came to the United States from Germany in the 1880s. His grandfather, Adolph Volcker, stood 6 feet 4 inches, sported a handlebar mustache, and bequeathed to the family not only his height but also his Teutonic reserve and strict, conservative moral code. In 1930, when Paul Volcker, Jr. was 3 years old, his father became Teaneck's first town manager. The town was in such bad financial shape that Paul Sr. took on the additional job of town engineer for only $1 per year. Both parents were devoted to their children but emotionally aloof. Paul Sr. held himself to the highest standards of public service, refusing any public action that might bring personal gain. When the chief of public works sent a plow to clear the family's driveway after a heavy snowstorm, Volcker told him never to do it again. When the principal at Teaneck High School put 15 high school seniors on the payroll as safety monitors and Paul Jr.'s name was on the list, his father saw nepotism. The principal was promptly fired.

Shy, quiet, and athletic, Volcker graduated from Teaneck High School at the top of his class. He went to Princeton University in the 1940s, intimidated by the school's reputation and surprised that he, a strong but unexceptional student from New Jersey, had been accepted at such an elite institution. Nevertheless, Volcker flourished academically, graduating from Princeton and earning financial assistance to Harvard University's Littauer School of

Public Administration, which later became the John F. Kennedy School of Government. He received a master's degree from Harvard in 1950 and spent a year abroad at the London School of Economics.

In 1952, Volcker joined the staff of the Federal Reserve Bank of New York as a full-time economist. Back home in New Jersey, he met Barbara Bahnson, the daughter of a general practitioner from Jersey City. They were married in 1954. At the time, as a young employee making $3,000 per year at the Fed, Volcker didn't have high hopes for the future. He told Barbara that he would never amount to much—that, probably, he would end up working in some dim office as an economist making a paltry salary.

In 1962, Robert Roosa, who had been his mentor at the Federal Reserve, hired Volcker at the Treasury Department. Almost two decades later, Volcker was named Chairman of the Federal Reserve—a job that saddled him with the responsibility for taming the soaring inflation that was sweeping the country. Volcker's unorthodox strategy was to make borrowing so expensive that individuals and businesses wouldn't take out new money for investment. This "tight money" strategy prompted harsh criticism.

By 1981, on the eve of Ronald Reagan's presidency, Volcker's policies had proved successful. A 1986 poll named Volcker second only to Reagan as the most influential person in the United States. Despite professional success, Volcker's 8-year tenure as chairman of the Fed was not a joyous experience for his family. Never motivated by personal material gain, he had accepted a $57,000 salary—more than a $50,000 pay cut from his previous job—and had to relocate to Washington, DC.

Meanwhile, Volcker's wife Barbara had long been suffering from the painful and crippling disease rheumatoid arthritis and stayed behind in New York. Volcker lived and worked in Washington during the week and on most weekends joined Barbara in New York. In 1987, with professional responsibilities taking an ever-larger toll on his family, Volcker resigned his position as Chairman of the Federal Reserve.

As we talk in his office, Volcker's comments suggest that he feels underused and out of place. I ask if he looks forward to working on new projects. "Yes, in theory, no in practice." We both chuckle. "I don't really want to get involved in something that's too big a project." But Volcker does have an idea that is important, if unsexy. He wants to create a new Institute for Public Administration, something he clearly learned first at his father's knee in Teaneck.

He hasn't been able to interest funders, political leaders, or universities. "People say, 'I don't know what public administration is, I'm not interested.'" Volcker thinks that all levels of government lack the knowledge, experience, and expertise to carry out their functions, a problem that later intensified during the Trump administration. He thinks people need more training and accountability. The heyday of public administration in the 1960s at schools such as Harvard or The University of Texas has long since faded. Endowments and funding now flow to schools of foreign policy and public policy.

"What's the difference between public policy and public administration?" I ask him.

"Public policy is big ideas. Everybody's in favor of public policy. You hire all kinds of people who want to write essays on that and they'll do op-ed pieces and an occasional book and so forth." Here, Volcker is getting really worked up. He met last week with the new president of the World Bank, who was complaining that no one was following up or implementing policies.

"So this is the kind of thing that gets your blood up," I say. He nods. Volcker applies this standard of efficiency and expertise to every level of government. "Do something simple," he says,

> Want to have an effective police department? That's a problem of public administration. You want to have effective budgeting in the state and get your accounts straight and have transparency and all the rest? . . . Go get it done. That's the hard work.

"It's one answer to the question of what would make you feel needed?"

"That's exactly right," he answers "I can give you a piece of paper that describes what I'd like to do, but do I have the energy to do it at this point is the question. Also I am constitutionally unable to ask for money."

"What does it mean in general to be needed?" I ask.

"There's a meaning to your life, I guess." Volcker hesitates. "It's a kind of selfish thing to say you want to be needed."

"No, everybody says that—everybody needs to be needed," I say. "I believe that."

"I'm sure you do, but it is kind of a selfish thought. Why do you think people think it's important that you be needed? Go home, go to sleep. You're dead, you're out of it, you're . . . we don't need you."

"What does that mean?" I ask.

"You may feel that you want to be needed," he says, "but the people in charge don't need you, they—I mean, people that need you are the people that are unhappy with something. So, you will start this new thing, but if you're a government official you don't want me—you don't want this old guy around.

At age 85, Volcker's body isn't what it used to be. His heart beats irregularly. His knees are bad. Although he has hearing aids in both ears, they don't solve all his problems. "That's what kills you," he says,

> You're making a speech in public or something. A woman gets up and asks a long question—I don't have the vaguest idea of what she is talking about. "I'm sorry, I can't hear you," I tell her. And then she talks a little louder and maybe a little more slowly and I begin to get half a clue.

When I tell Volcker that I'm interested in his idea of manhood—especially his experience of sexuality—we play a bit of a cat-and-mouse game.

"It's a category that you wish you could perform more vigorously, yes," he says.

"Yeah, tell me about that."

"I cannot tell you," he laughs.

"Typically we think about male midlife and Viagra and sexual performance. Is that still a concern for you?"

"It's more an annoyance, I guess. . . . No, it's a great concern. You really feel that you're less than a full man."

"Sure," I say. "Do you think that's a common but unexpressed thought?"

"It must be."

I can't believe that I'm actually talking to the former Chairman of the Federal Reserve about his sex life. "I really appreciate your honesty," I say. "There aren't many people willing to talk about that. What about other aspects of being a man?"

"I worry about the future of mankind," he says. "The women are demanding more and more and more. And if the women get half the good jobs in the world, what the hell are the men going to end up doing?"

It takes me a minute to understand that Volcker is literally worried about the future of "man-kind." "If women have all the same ambitions as men and are successful," Volker says, "what's that mean for men? I don't know, men will be digging the ditches or something." I realize that Volcker isn't entirely joking.

For a minute or two, Volcker and I spar over this issue. Although we disagree, I think he does put his finger on interesting and important questions: What are men for? What kind of man will take his place alongside the new kind of woman emerging in the 21st century? Volcker could well have been reading Hanna Rosin's *The End of Men: And the Rise of Women*. In that book, whose title is exaggerated for effect, Rosin highlights the economic shift which Volcker refers to. In the Great Recession that followed the financial crisis of 2008, men lost three-fourths of the 7.5 million jobs that disappeared. The loss of work in typically male industries—construction, manufacturing, and high finance—was accompanied by a rise in women's education, workforce participation, and income. More than half the American workforce now consists of women, who outnumber men in colleges and professional schools and are becoming the breadwinners in increasingly more families. Approximately 80% of women aged 25–54 years work for pay. Whereas women held 26% of managerial and professional jobs in 1980, by 2011, they held more than 50% of them.

In the new postindustrial economy, which values typically "female" attributes such as empathy, patience, communication, and problem-solving, women have adapted more quickly than men. Despite this progress, women still do not receive equal pay for equal work; still experience discrimination; and, as was increasingly revealed after 2016, face a staggering amount of sexual harassment.

"So this is a genuine concern for you?" I ask.

"Yeah, it's a genuine concern. It's not going to happen to me, but I just kind of wonder. 50 years from now you'll probably have a revolt of the men. Now I've identified myself as a weird, masculine . . ."

"You're entitled to your regressive social views," I laugh. "You're one of our most esteemed male leaders."

Volcker wonders what the man of the future will be like. "You can answer that question," he says. "You're a young man."

In 1967, when I entered all-male Yale College, we wore gray flannel suits and ties to freshman orientation, where President Kingman Brewster reminded us of the importance of a liberal education and our duty to become leaders. I'll never forget the hilarious foretaste of feisty feminism I witnessed that day. Professor Trinkaus, a biologist known for demeaning women as well as his fondness of alcohol, was giving a talk when he noticed a female graduate student knitting in the front row.

"You know," he said, "Knitting is a form of masturbation."

"You do it your way and I'll do it mine," she answered.

When I was a freshman, Yale was known as an institution whose mission was to graduate "1,000 male leaders" every year. We got drunk from silver bowls at Mory's famous drinking club, swam naked at the pools in the Payne Whitney Gymnasium, and took for granted the privileges of being men at an elite Ivy League school. When Yale accepted women undergraduates for the first time in 1969, we enjoyed the gifts of new romances and faced the challenges of in-your-face feminism. In "consciousness-raising groups," we sat together in our dorm rooms and discussed equal pay for work, equal access to education and employment, the gendered division of labor in the household, and the ways that devaluing women was built into our everyday language and jokes. It wasn't easy to be a target in those discussions, where the idea of women's equality in my head did not always match the assumptions of privilege and superiority in my heart. And by the 1970s, our liberal arts education, together with Western humanism and the "rights of man," would come under fire as little more than the ideas of dead white men.

Volcker is correct about feminism's influence on me. But I also know that he's baiting me, so I decide to play along.

"You're on the wrong side of history," I say.

"Don't be so sure," he answers. "What will it mean to be a man? We'll be the linemen for the telephone company going up the telephone pole. Why do women want to do that too? I really wonder."

I tell Volcker a bit about my personal view of manhood, which includes a fluid transition between gender roles, support for women's work outside the household, a commitment to mutual decision-making, and a personality in which emotion is not segregated from intellect.

"What does that mean?" he asks.

"I don't know. I'm interviewing you," I say. "We should sit down and have a drink over this."

I ask Volcker how his questions apply to older men. "If you're old enough, it doesn't make any difference," he answers, meaning that the worst of gender equality was still in the future.

In some ways, Volcker embodies an older, patrician vision of manhood—a moral code that takes male dominance for granted and at the same time values community and character. Even as he worries about the future of "mankind," Volcker inhabits his current patriarchal role comfortably, without question.

I wonder what Volcker is afraid of. "Are you afraid of death?" I ask.

Not particularly. Not at this stage, anyway—my sister just died a year or so ago and she was a little bit older than I was, and she was quite active. She was 85, and she got cancer and went down pretty fast, in a year or so. It was interesting. She didn't want to go through the agony of cancer treatment. She thought: "I don't care whether I live 2 more years. When my time has come, it's come."

"I don't know," Volcker continues,

I hope I feel that way at some point when I get really sick. I don't sit around worrying about dying. You do wonder whether you're going to get a heart attack or something once in a while, like in my case you get a stroke—my father died from a stroke. It's crazy. I thought he was an old man—he was 70. You don't think of a 70-year-old being an old man anymore. My mother was 68 when my father died. She lived another 30 years.

When Volcker retired from the Federal Reserve, he thought he'd find a short-term job and retire in a few years. It was not an easy time.

I was 60. I had no money, I had a sick wife, I had a handicapped son, I had a daughter who is self-sufficient, but she was a nurse at that point—she wasn't going to be rich. I said okay, I'm 60, I came out of a prominent position and obviously I can get a job someplace, I've got 5 years to make some money because people retire at 65. When 5 years were up I got so goddam busy I couldn't keep up with it.

Now he's sitting here, 25 years later, still at work. I mention to Volcker that he didn't tell me what he's afraid of.

I'm afraid of not being able to hear. I'm afraid of having a stroke like my father. And everybody's afraid of Alzheimer's. I got a real problem—I can't remember people's names anymore. I was never good at remembering people's names, but now it's really bad.

It's almost 3 o'clock. Anke, Volcker's longtime administrator, executive secretary, and constant companion—now his wife—opens the door and signals that it's time for Volcker's next appointment. Paul Volcker is not a man given to speculation or introspection or personal revelation, certainly not with strangers or interviewers. Anke's appearance snaps him back to his public persona.

"Why am I talking to you like this? You're insidious!"

"I'm a good listener," I say, turning off the recorder.

## CHAPTER 7

Denton Cooley and the Legacy
of 100,000 Hearts

In 1969, Dr. Denton Cooley implanted the first artificial heart in a human being and soon after became the first American to perform a heart transplant. Throughout the years, he became one of the most famous surgeons on the planet. Cooley's accomplishments are stunning: He pioneered the heart–lung machine that made open-heart surgery possible, helped develop a method to repair torn aortic aneurysms, was at one point the world's authority on congenital heart defects in children, and was an early advocate of coronary artery bypass graft for treating blocked blood vessels. When his assistant didn't respond to my request for an interview in the summer of 2013, I had assumed that 93-year-old Cooley had other things to do with his time. Several months later, I received an apology explaining that she had misplaced my email and that Dr. Cooley would be happy to visit with me.

Cooley works in a wavy 10-story building that contains operating rooms, offices, rooms for patient bed care, laboratories, a 500-seat auditorium for telemedicine, conference rooms, rooms for teaching, a museum, a videotaping studio, and a helipad. It is of course the Denton A. Cooley Building. My office is less than half a mile away in the Jesse Jones Library, a 4-story building that opens onto one of the few remaining green spaces in the Texas Medical Center (TMC), the largest medical complex in the world. It's difficult to convey the size of the TMC, a loose association of approximately 60 institutions that collectively employ more than 100,000 people who see 8 million patients per year. Its major institutions are in a perpetual building frenzy, each one competing to construct the tallest building or to display the flashiest logo. The prize undoubtedly goes to MD Anderson Cancer Center, whose buildings metastasize faster than the cancer it works to cure.

Much of the Jesse H. Jones Library building, built in 1954, is barely usable. The elevators are so old and unreliable that when I set out to meet Dr. Cooley, I decide to take the stairs. Unfortunately, walking with my arthritic hip is barely more reliable than using the elevators.

Waiting for the elevator inside the Texas Heart Institute, I struggle with my own smallness. There is probably not a single question to which Cooley doesn't have prefabricated answers—except, I realize, questions about being an old man. So I am surprised by his openness to the topic and by his generosity toward me. Cooley's legendary ruthless and competitive spirit have obviously softened. He gives me a copy of his recently published memoir, *100,000 Hearts*, and inscribes it "To Thomas Cole, Ph.D. With warm regards and gratitude for his interest in my life. Denton Cooley."

Cooley speaks slowly, with a slight Texas twang, sometimes slurring his words. He has retained most of his wavy hair, now white and parted on the left. His cheeks are still full, his nose strong and handsome. "Everything seems to revolve around my coming to the hospital and to my office," Cooley tells me,

> and I look forward to it. I get up every morning at 6:30 or 7:00, have coffee and take medications and visit with my wife and read parts of the morning paper. I usually leave home about 7:30 and drive myself to the hospital.

For decades as a working surgeon with the fastest hands in the business, Cooley drove to work before sunrise, returned after sundown, and often made another trip to see a patient or two in the middle of the night. These days he meets with his business manager once a week to oversee his investments and his children's trust funds. He is determined not to repeat the embarrassing bankruptcy he filed at the age of 67, when Houston real estate prices plummeted along with the price of oil.

In a long life that has revolved around professional activities, some things—like coming to the office every day—haven't changed. But other things, like getting from one building to the next, require some help. "I have an electric chair—an electric scooter," Cooley says, "which I use to get around the hospital. And then I come to my office and begin my day's activities."

At age 93, Cooley worries about losing his independence, his good looks, and his mental abilities. What man doesn't share this same vulnerability of lapsing into a second childhood? In Cooley's case, these fears seem especially intense. He and his wife Louise refuse to go to assisted living, and their house has been rearranged to accommodate their serious physical limitations.

A decade ago, when he underwent surgery for colon cancer, Cooley stopped operating on patients. His daughter Susan became worried about her father's mental health and asked his colleague Bernard Levin at MD Anderson Cancer Center for advice. "Here's what you do," he told Susan. "You send him back to work. You call all of his friends and colleagues and you make sure that they visit him. Do not put him out to pasture." Susan followed Levin's advice, and Cooley's mood improved.

Today, even though he drives to work and zips along the hospital's hallways on his motorized scooter, Cooley still wonders whether he matters. "So many old people get depressed," he tells me. "And I must confess that I get depressed, too."

I ask Cooley how he responds during these moments. "I try to give myself some psychiatric treatment," he says. "I tell myself, 'this is not how you want to end your footrace. It would detract significantly from your legacy.'"

Ever the competitor, Cooley thinks of himself as a marathon runner. Of course, whenever Cooley crosses the finish line, he will no longer be around to worry. And he needn't. Like other men of his age and eminence, Cooley is continuously asked to accept honors and awards at fundraising events. Cooley doesn't chafe at his honorary status. He enjoys it. He is a generous donor to institutions for renovations or buildings that bear his name. Unlike Paul Volcker, he doesn't yearn to be in charge anymore. Instead, Cooley seems most concerned with the fragility of his legacy, as if a strand of his light blue cardigan sweater might come loose at any moment and unravel the whole thing.

When I ask Cooley what he regrets, he mentions the infamous 40-year dispute and rivalry with Michael DeBakey, the equally accomplished heart surgeon who also lived and practiced in Houston at Baylor College of Medicine and the Veterans Affairs Medical Center. "Everybody knew Mike DeBakey," Cooley tells me. "It was a household name, and then to establish a rivalry with this man—I think that helped my career enormously."

"Competition is a good thing," I agree.

Cooley nods. "I've always told some of my younger trainees, 'Look, if the opportunity comes along for you to develop a rivalry with some person in surgery or medicine, pick somebody who is up high. Don't pick somebody down low.'"

In the late 1960s, many researchers, Cooley included, hoped that a total artificial heart (TAH) would be the next major breakthrough in cardiac surgery. By most accounts, Cooley stole the first artificial heart—and the fame that came with it—from DeBakey, precipitating a long and bitter feud. But Cooley tells a different story in his autobiography *100,000 Hearts*. According to him, Domingo Liotta, an Argentinian surgeon, repeatedly attempted to contact DeBakey for help. Since Liotta never got a response, he finally went to see DeBakey in person and showed him a prototype of the artificial heart. Barely glancing at it, DeBakey told Liotta never to bother him about it again.

Liotta and Cooley began collaborating. Both of them believed that the TAH was ready for human use in a desperate situation. Among several patients who were awaiting cardiac transplantation, Haskell Karp was in perhaps the poorest shape. The TAH, Cooley believed, was the only thing that might save Karp's life. He went ahead with the procedure. The transplanted heart worked well at first, but Karp's weak immune system led to renal failure and acute pneumonia in his right lung. He died just 32 hours after the transplant.

Although Mr. Karp lost his heroic struggle, Cooley was convinced that a TAH could work as a bridge to transplantation. DeBakey was enraged that Cooley hadn't requested his permission to go through with the transplant. News of the TAH implant, which DeBakey received from the morning papers, led to their complete break. "In a newspaper interview," Cooley recalls, "he claimed that the operation was a 'stunt' that had no useful research purpose. According to Mike, the only reason I had performed the operation was because I wanted to be the first. Both statements were false."

"In the months after the TAH transplant," Cooley continues,

I called Mike several times and left messages but never got a response. In fact, he would not speak to me again for nearly forty years. If we happened to attend the same medical meeting, he would act as if I didn't exist.

The two surgeons finally reconciled in 2007 in a series of public displays, one of which fittingly served as a fundraiser for the Texas Heart Institute. I was in attendance that night at the Houston Country Club, and I remember the pleasure of those whose hearts were warmed and whose pocketbooks were opened.

Aside from the infamous "feud," our conversation touches on two of Cooley's other regrets. In 1985, Cooley's 28-year-old daughter Florence was found dead in her apartment from an apparently self-inflicted gunshot wound to the head. "Florence's death was the worst tragedy of my life," he says,

The sadness was overwhelming. Not only do I miss her terribly, but I feel like I failed her. I continue to ask myself whether I could have done more to help her—maybe somehow treated her differently, so that she wouldn't have taken that final, desperate step.

Cooley's belated feelings of guilt reflect the price younger generations often pay for their parent's greatness. At the time, Cooley was at the height of his fame and success. Looking back now, he wonders, "Maybe I just wasn't there enough for her."

Cooley also regrets the bankruptcy that followed his daughter's suicide. In the 1980s, as one of Houston's elites, he enjoyed all the outward signs of success—the pillared mansion, the charity benefits, Rolls Royces decorating his driveway. *Forbes Magazine* estimated the Texas surgeon–businessman's net worth to be approximately $40 million and growing. But then something surprising happened: In 1987, Cooley filed for Chapter 11 bankruptcy. As an amateur investor who had ventured into real estate, he had borrowed and spent millions on office buildings and apartment complexes during the oil boom. When plummeting oil prices pulled the rug out from under Houston and the rest of the oil patch economy, Cooley suddenly owed $100 million. "And here I was," he says with chagrin, "perceived as not only a great surgeon, but also a financial genius, a huge success, an athlete, someone who does everything well."

The most devastating effect of the bankruptcy was that it threatened the image of success Cooley had fashioned himself. *100,000 Hearts*, for example, is filled with images of a healthy, athletic, successful Denton Cooley—by the beach, at the golf course, on the tennis or basketball court. Other photos feature him alongside family; friends; colleagues; and even Presidents Ronald Reagan, Bill Clinton, and George H. W. Bush.

I ask Cooley what else worries him about being old.

"Well, every old guy worries about his bowels," Cooley says. "Most everything revolves around when and if your bowels are going to move." Losing control of his bowels, soiling or wetting himself, is an especially frightening prospect to Cooley, a man who has devoted his life to repairing, managing, and controlling the human body. It would constitute a failure and a source of deep shame.

Although he won't give it up, Cooley also worries about his driving. "Some people wonder whether a 93-year-old is entitled to have a driver's license," Cooley said,

but I don't know what I would do without that opportunity. And every now and then I come close to an accident or I might not see a pedestrian crossing in front of my car. And something like that would just be a real tragedy to me.

I worry about his driving too. A year or so before our conversation, I was walking to a celebratory event at the University of Texas Dental School. It was dark outside. An old man sped out of the parking lot in a black Cadillac and almost ran me over. It was Cooley.

Denton Cooley died on November 18, 2016. About a year later, his daughter Susan, a nurse and a former faculty member, came to visit with me about collaborative teaching possibilities. On the spur of the moment, I asked if she'd talk with me about the last years of her parents' lives, when she supervised their care and medical decision-making. Although the memories were still raw, she agreed. She began by talking about her mother.

During at least the last decade of her life, Louise Cooley suffered from anemia and terribly painful rheumatoid arthritis. Yet, Susan says, "she was absolutely committed to caring for my father, managing the last years of his life, and caring for him at the end." They lived in a plantation-style Southern colonial house on a quarter-acre of land in Houston's exclusive River Oaks neighborhood. In those years, Cooley slept downstairs in his modified office because he couldn't get up the stairs to the second floor.

Even in her 90s, in the face of excruciating pain, Louise woke up every morning at 6 a.m., rode her motorized chair down the stairs, had breakfast with her husband, and took him to his car. After he drove to work, she would go back upstairs where she rested and got organized for the day so that she'd be ready when Cooley came home. "He'd call and say, 'I'm on my way,'" Susan remembers. "She rode that scooter thing back down the stairs to be ready for dinner and the evening when he got home." Then they went to sleep in their separate bedrooms.

One night while she was going to the bathroom, Louise fell and couldn't get up. Cooley heard her calling out and managed to get upstairs. He reached down to help her stand up and fell down himself. When Susan arrived the next morning, her parents were lying next to each other on the bathroom floor, holding hands.

Toward the end of her life, Louise was in excruciating pain and became increasingly frail. The oxygen levels in her blood kept falling, and she required regular blood transfusions. Louise's hematologist and Susan and Cooley wondered about continuing the transfusions, which seemed to accomplish little beyond extending Louise's suffering. When Susan told Louise that it might be time to discontinue treatment, Louise asked, "Do you want me to die?"

"She was upset because her plan was that he was going to die first," Susan says,

Because that was her job. It never occurred to anybody that she would go first. That just wasn't in the plan. They always joked. My mother would say, "Well, what do you want for your funeral?" "Surprise me" was his answer.

As her mother's anemia got worse, Susan decided that Cooley needed to talk to Louise before any decision was made. Cooley had no capacity to have discussions about end-of-life issues. He didn't want any Do Not Resuscitate orders for her, didn't even want to say the word "hospice," and didn't want to talk to his wife about any of it. But Susan was insistent:

> I called my father and said, "Today is the day that you are going to talk to your wife. You're going to do it." And he said, "Well, what am I going to say?" And so I coached him through what to say. When he came home he had obviously been struggling, struggling, struggling with this. And he walked in the back-door, just with this downtrodden face. And he pulled this little scrap of paper out of his pocket, and on it in his jittery handwriting, it said, "Dilemma." And he had written out the definition: "a problem for which there are two equally bad solutions." And so I took him upstairs, sat him next to her bed, put his hand on hers, whispered in his ear what to say.

"What did you tell him?" I ask.

"We need to have a conversation. And I love you. I think it's time we stop doing this. And what that's going to mean is you'll go to sleep. And this is really hard."

"What happened?" I ask.

"He couldn't do it. And he said everything except for that. And he said, 'So do you want to keep having your blood transfusions?' She said, 'Yes.'"

"Why couldn't he tell her?" I ask.

"He was too sad. He knew we weren't going to give her any more blood transfusions."

Tears well up in Susan's eyes. Her voice trails off:

> I mean, she was getting worse and worse and worse with the pain and—it was merciful. We could've kept her alive. But we would be carrying her around on a stretcher. It was a huge moral dilemma. Three-quarters of me knows that it was right. The other quarter knows that I robbed her of her autonomy, her desire to stay alive, to be in charge of him, which was her life.

"At the end," Susan remembers, "all he said to her was 'Well, we'll see.' And then he got up and left."

Without another blood transfusion, Louise Cooley slipped into a coma. Cooley refused to allow hospice into their home. So Susan brought in other caregivers. As Louise lay dying, Susan and her sisters, Mary, "Weezie," and Helen, gathered around the bed. When Susan started to bring her father upstairs to be present when Louise died, one of the caregivers pulled her aside and said it would be better to let Cooley stay downstairs, to spare him the pain of watching his wife die. "She told me, 'Go ahead and let her die and get her cleaned up and then let him come up and see her.' And it was the right thing."

I pause for a few moments to let Susan catch her breath. And then I ask, "So how did your father go?"

"He probably had a pulmonary embolism [a blocked artery in the lungs] at home," she answers. Cooley had decided that he would never go to hospice or back to the hospital. For a week or two, he sat in his chair or lay in bed. Episodes of pain or difficulty breathing filled the nights. "The caregivers called me over two or three times a week in the middle of the night—it was like having a new baby some weeks." At approximately 5 a.m. one morning, Susan was at the bedside when Dr. Carl Dahlberg, a pulmonary and critical care physician, walked in. "He listened to my father's lungs, and he said, 'Yeah he's got pneumonia.' And I said, 'Well, we're not going to treat him, are we?' And he said, 'Good. That's what I wanted to say.'"

After a few days, Cooley began hallucinating. A colleague told Susan that these were terminal hallucinations and that the drug Haldol might ease his agitation. Instead, she says, it made him more belligerent. After they stopped the Haldol, Cooley turned to Susan and told her that she had to call an ambulance. "We had a pact that he would never go to the hospital," she says. "So I asked him, 'Do you really want to go to the hospital?' 'No, I want to go home. I want to go home. I want to go home,' he said." Cooley had spent so much of his life in the hospital that Susan wondered, "what home did he want to go to? He kept saying 'dial this phone number,' and it was the hospital phone number."

Cooley soon slipped into a coma. His children came and gathered around him. After several days, Susan and Dr. Dahlberg began wondering why Cooley was not actively dying. "Carl couldn't figure it out," she says. "And then he said, 'Uh-oh. He has a pacemaker!'" Susan chuckles as she tells the story. "We called the pacemaker guy, who was just pulling out of his driveway in the morning."

One month to the day after Louise Cooley's death, that pacemaker technician came over and turned off the heart of the most famous heart surgeon in the world.

| John Harper Gets by with a Little Help from His Friends

After driving through lush green fields of shoulder-high corn, I reach a small bluff and turn into John Harper's driveway in Iowa City, Iowa. His blue one-story 1960s ramshackle ranch house is in various states of repair and disrepair. Harper arrives at the front door in a short-sleeved, blue-green plaid shirt worn above a black T-shirt, grayish canvas shorts, and suede moccasins. His smile is easy and his belly rotund. We sit at the kitchen table eating the stale white-bread tuna sandwiches and pasta salad he'd picked up for lunch.

Harper is a 76-year-old gay man, ailing yet vital, whose life has touched literary luminaries such as Tennessee Williams, Kurt Vonnegut, Anthony Burgess, and Arthur Miller. He isn't someone who has won prestigious awards for writing or performance or preaching. Instead, he's slyly accomplished in ways that link him to powerful people and make everyone around him better. His life is a story of deep friendships that zigzags across work, play, and community life. As ever, Harper's schedule is crammed. Tonight is a rehearsal for the musical revue in which he is performing for a local charity. Born in March 1941 to strict Disciples of Christ parents, Harper started in finance after earning an undergraduate degree at Stanford University. He seems to have lived three different lives: as an administrator and then a professor at the University of Iowa's prestigious English Department; as an Episcopal priest and co-founder of New Song Church in nearby Coralville; and as founder, actor, and director of a local community theater. Harper served in so many organizations and on so many boards that Governor Robert Ray honored him with the Iowa Community Betterment Award.

Early in our conversation, a chipmunk darts across the screened-in porch adjacent to the kitchen. Harper gets up, looks at the creature kindly, and closes the sliding glass door. "He'll find his own way out," he says. It's as if the chipmunk is his neighbor, like the chirping birds or the handyman who came to repair his driveway. I envy the small-town ease and closeness to nature of John's daily life. Yet his house feels lonely to me.

Harper is a charismatic and vulnerable man. He mostly avoids my eyes by looking upward or swiveling his head first to the right and then to the left. Occasionally, he shoots me a searching glance to see if I'm following him. I am. My steady gaze is meant to hold him securely through whatever he needs to say, for however long it takes. For the first 2 hours, Harper is ebullient, funny, and eager to recount his zigzagging life.

In 1967, when he was 26 years old, Harper came out as a gay man. It was an act of courage in an America that was virulently anti-gay. Only 2 years earlier, at the Stonewall uprising in Greenwich Village, gay men fought back against a police raid aimed at dispersing or arresting them. Under the repressive anti-communist regime of the 1950s and 1960s, gay men, lesbians, and transgender people were on the list of groups considered to be national security risks (a thin disguise for violent prejudice). Police broke up gatherings, shut down gay bars, and arrested gay customers and printed their names in newspapers. Universities expelled instructors they suspected of being homosexuals. The American Psychiatric Association classified homosexuality as a form of mental illness—a classification that wasn't removed until 1973. Individuals we now consider members of LGBTQ communities were physically harassed, humiliated, fired, jailed, or sent to mental hospitals. To avoid such treatment, many led double lives.

I ask Harper what it was like to claim his sexual identity in those days.

"You pretty much knew nobody who was gay and out," he says. "There were no resources—nobody knew what 'gay' meant. People thought: 'This is a man who really wanted to be a woman.' That's about how much was known."

Harper didn't only suffer from cultural ignorance and prejudice. He also had his heart broken. "I fell in love hard a couple of times and had very intense relationships with men who then went off and married women and had children," he tells me. "It's taken a lifetime to kind of forgive that and to realize that they did the only thing they could imagine doing. That was how the world worked."

I ask if he still felt the pain of those relationships.

I'll tell you where the pain comes most intensely—getting reconnected with those early great loves and hearing: "The time I was with you is the only time in my life I was ever truly happy." And I think, "Thanks a lot for saying this fifty years later, dumb ass."

Although none of Harper's early gay relationships survived and matured, he's worked tirelessly on behalf of gay and lesbian causes in the church, the academy, the theater, and the community. "John inhabits the ship of his own beliefs and will sail into a storm if he has to," says Rick McCarthy, a gay minister, theologian, and John's former student. He continues,

John was often attracted to people, and he didn't shy away from others' attraction to him. He took the message of the gospel in Peter—"nothing I have made is impure"—to mean that acts are only made impure on the inside, in one's heart.

Harper's sexuality, says McCarthy, was voracious. Despite the recent separation of sex and love in much of America, mainstream culture still views short sexual encounters—especially gay arousal and orgasm—as morally wrong. Harper, on the other hand, viewed his brief and intense sexual encounters as holy relationships characterized by mutual caring and consent.

I ask if sexuality is still a part of his personal life.

"I would say not."

"Is that a regret?"

"It is. But it's kind of irreversible. I had prostate cancer surgery in 2004. They told me that beyond that I would not really be so interested in sex anymore. Wrong!"

Sex is possible with great difficulty. Orgasm is not. I miss that. Every once in a while, I think about how much I took for granted. It does pop into my head from time to time that orgasm and erection is more of a manhood issue than being gay is.

"Does that mean you feel that you're less of a man if you can't have an erection?"

There's a tiny bit of that. I wouldn't say I ever obsess on it, but yeah. You know I have in my stable of friendships so much gender fluidity going on that I'm not sure trying to identify what is masculinity and what is femininity really accomplishes anything.

Harper tells me about a young friend of his who started the first gay Greek fraternity on campus at the University of Iowa. One evening, Harper and his friend went to dinner to celebrate the university's sanctioning of the new fraternity. They talked for hours. Sitting at the table and viewed from the waist up, Harper's friend looked like a heterosexual, masculine frat boy. "It was only when we were out the door and starting down the sidewalk," Harper says,

> that I saw he was wearing six-inch heels and Capri pants. When we got downtown, all of the jocks and the typical frat boys were hitting the bar. I've never seen anything like the verbal abuse heaped on him as we walked down the street.

After an hour and a half, Harper excuses himself. Soon I do the same. When I get to the bathroom, I notice cobwebs spanning a corner of the dusty floorboards at my feet. Maybe the spiders are trying to span the separated walls of Harper's life.

Friendship is a seriously undervalued dimension of love and meaning among older people. It is especially important for gay men in John's generation, when gay marriage was not legal and gay and lesbian couples raising children was unheard of. After our conversation in Iowa City, I spoke by phone with four of Harper's friends who come from the distinct silos of his life. In addition to Rick McCarthy, I talked to Elizabeth Coulter, who founded the New Song Episcopal Church with John in 1994; Penelope Hall, who has worked with him in community theater since the 1970s; and Dee Morris, John's colleague who came out as a lesbian and later became Chair of the Department of English at the University of Iowa. John's deep friends barely know each other. And yet they all stress his steadfast presence as a mentor, colleague, and friend.

John has long been a source of inspiration and encouragement for Rick McCarthy. Years ago, when McCarthy was stressed out preparing for his last graduate school exams, John met him at a Perkins pancake house. At the table, John's gaze often swiveled past Rick's, as if he were looking out a window into the story of his life. Then he looked searchingly back at Rick and said, "Sometimes you feel like the greatest fraud, don't you?"

In a strange way, John's words were exactly what Rick needed to hear: an affirmation that, even as he was trying to become an expert in his field, no one can ever be the ultimate authority on a subject. Rick passed his exams, got an academic job, and earned tenure. All the while, John was there for him.

John also needed Rick. When one of John's friends passed away from AIDS, he told Rick that he was too upset to go to the funeral by himself. So

Rick came to Iowa City to comfort John. "To sit there and be a presence was a gift to him," he said.

Harper lived his academic life in the University of Iowa's English Department, where he started out as an administrator and was later invited to teach as an assistant professor. "My first experiences teaching in the college classroom were high points," he tells me,

> I cut my teeth on the teaching profession right at the end of the 60s, as the whole world was exploding. And nothing about a class period was the slightest bit predictable. I might walk in and say, all right today we're going to discuss the principal aspects of symbolism in Conrad's *Heart of Darkness*. Someone in the third row would yell, "Like hell we are!" and someone in the fifth row would yell, "Fuck that! Don't you know there's a war going on?" In the back rows there are joints being passed up and down the rows. And very often I had to walk through picket lines just to get into my own classroom building.

As a radical student myself in the late 1960s and early 1970s, I could have been one of John's students, often traveling to Washington, DC, for anti-war rallies, being buzzed by army helicopters while camping out on the National Mall and gassed by Washington riot police on horseback breaking up one of our rallies at the Justice Department.

"We thought the whole world was watching," I say. Harper nods.

Despite radical student rebellion, the English Department at the University of Iowa became a flourishing literary center. Planted amid Midwestern cornfields, far from prestigious coastal universities, the English Department was the first program in the country to accept fiction and poetry as a PhD thesis. By John's time, the department's Iowa Writers' Workshop had become the leading creative writing program in the country. When we talked—more than 15 years after his retirement—he was writing an authorized history of the English department from the 1920s to the present.

In characteristic fashion, John didn't pursue the standard path of a scholar diligently publishing his or her way to the status of senior professor. Instead, he embraced teaching and cultivated personal relationships with many students and writers. Two students in the program, John Irving and Gail Godwin, became famous writers. John was a regular in the Iowa Writers' Workshop poker game, where he met visiting faculty such as Kurt Vonnegut, the author of *Slaughterhouse Five*; novelist Anthony Burgess, who wrote *A Clockwork Orange*; and playwright Tennessee Williams, whose *Cat on a Hot Tin Roof* became one of John's favorite plays.

When Dee Morris arrived at the University of Iowa English Department in 1974, she quickly recognized John as a well-liked and influential faculty member. In the 1980s, Morris left her husband and came out as a lesbian. At a time when many faculty treated her as a pariah, Harper stood with her in solidarity. "I could feel his support and I could feel his own pain," she told me.

During the next 30 years, American culture's hostility toward gay people began to soften. In 2009, John—by then an Episcopal minister—gracefully orchestrated the interfaith marriage between Dee, a Jew, and her wife Wendy, a Buddhist. At the end of that ceremony, people in the audience—many of whom had long been hostile to their relationship—leapt to their feet in applause. "John was there for us," Dee said. "It was a joyful moment."

Dee Morris admired John as a kind of "number two man"—an eccentric, creative, behind-the-scenes operator who made programs and people better. Despite academics who resented him for carving out a unique path, John wielded considerable influence. He played a key role in establishing university programs in black studies, women's studies, sexuality studies, printing and design, and international literature. "Unlike most of us who move hesitantly from square to square," Dee said, likening academia to a board game, "John is the sort of player who sees six moves ahead, but even better, he's a player who nudges you to turn here, warns you not to go there, and rejoices when you get home safe."

Penelope Hall, a lifelong theater administrator, describes Harper as a bustling, easygoing man with a rare sense of humor. "He is an excellent theater director: really very very good, and it was a joy to work with him," she told me. John and Penelope were 2 of 18 founding members of the City Circle Acting Company, a theater group that was launched in 1984. Thanks to John's hard work and charisma—he served as the company's initial treasurer—the city of Coralville gave the group a brand new theater building. "It was really quite incredible," she said.

John's most memorable experience in theater took place in the summer of 1995, when he was invited to Alaska to work under the tutelage of Arthur Miller. Every summer, the University of Iowa theater program featured one playwright for its summer repertoire. Harper was asked to serve as a director. "You can imagine both the thrill and the terror of rehearsing and directing a scene from *Death of a Salesman* with Arthur Miller sitting there as my critic," Harper says laughing. "He was very kind to me, though."

Throughout the years, the City Circle Acting Company has performed a diverse collection of plays, including *Guys and Dolls, Hello Dolly!, A Christmas Carol, Our Town, The Hobbit,* and *Fiddler on the Roof.* And John is still acting—or trying to, when his body cooperates. Not long after we met at his house, Harper went to the grocery store after church one Sunday and tripped on a food crate. It was a nasty fall that put him out of commission for a few weeks.

All things considered, that fall was a relatively minor medical problem in a long series that includes hospitalizations, intensive chemotherapy, radiation, and surgery for recurring prostate cancer—not to mention coronary heart disease, arthritis, urinary leakage, and neuropathy. "I've decided that I'm the cash cow for the med center," he says.

Two winters before we met, Harper suffered his first heart attack and was taken to the emergency room at Desert Regional in Palm Springs, California:

> Because they were overcrowded and understaffed I just lay there in a little cubical all hooked up, and I looked at this heart monitor while the heart rate just went down and down and down—pretty soon it was getting into low forties, then into the thirties. And I said to myself, 'My God, this is it. The monitor is going all the way down to zero and then I'll be dead.'

That didn't happen, of course. But Harper's priest came to see him. They talked long into the night. The priest, seeing Harper so obviously troubled, asked what was bothering him. Harper answered that it was the fear of dying with half-finished manuscripts, dying without his life's work complete. At the same time, John's belief in an afterlife relieves the terror of total extinction.

Harper's religious life has complicated familial roots. Two of his great-grandfathers were early leaders in the Disciples of Christ church community in Des Moines, Iowa. As a young boy, John would take the bus to church alone and sit in the first row, mesmerized by an old Midwestern minister. His parents, who often partied hard on Saturday nights, snuck in late and sat at the back. Although his parents had little interest in church, Harper joined the Episcopal Cathedral in Des Moines, where he performed as a soloist in the boys' choir, fell in love with the liturgy, and felt called to the ministry. But year after year, decade after decade, Harper's ministerial aspirations were pushed aside in favor of other interests. He became impatient with the church's conservative positions on civil rights and the Vietnam War. He drifted away.

Harper was almost 50 years old when the call to ministry returned. At the time, in 1991, he was teaching at a university in southern France. He was lonely. With plenty of time to talk to himself and to God, he made a list of priorities: to think more seriously about ministry or a new career, to move out of his old-fashioned three-story Victorian house and dump all of his possessions, and to "divest" himself of his partner of approximately 6 years.

Sitting in Harper's worn-down house, I wince when he uses "divest" to describe plans for leaving his partner—as if his partner were some kind of financial entanglement. His choice of words suggests detached calculation rather than mutual commitment and emotional closeness.

When he returned home from France, Harper made good on all three decisions: He moved out of his house, left his partner, and trained to become ordained a deacon. But there was another complication: Gay ordination was deeply controversial in the Episcopal church. Becoming a deacon was not for the faint of heart. He was fortunate that Carl Christopher Epting, the newly appointed bishop of Iowa, supported his ordination while warning him of the opposition he'd face. "No outed gay has been ordained here," Epting told him. "It's not a fate I would wish on a dog, but if you'll agree to do it, I promise I'll be right by your side every step of the way."

Harper had nightmares of fights breaking out at his service—something that actually happened at an ordination service in New Hampshire. On the day of his ordination, the bishop reached the moment in the service when, as in a marriage ceremony, the officiant asks if anyone objects. The congregation was stone silent. No one coughed or moved. Then, for some reason, a member of the crowd giggled. Another giggled, and another. "Pretty soon half the place was just laughing their asses off," Harper says. "The bishop finally just kind of scratched his head and said: 'I assume that reaction means I can go ahead with this.'"

In 1992, Elizabeth Coulter was interning as a seminarian at Trinity Church in Iowa City. Harper, by then an Episcopal deacon, was also living a thrilling multifaceted life as a gay activist and adventurer. He would go out with friends dressed in drag and then, coming home the next morning, scurry to his bedroom to change for a faculty meeting—or for theater practice, or for class, or for church service. "I can't tell you the trust that people have for him," Coulter said of Harper's congregation. "They just trust him. They trust him to be hilarious and to make us laugh."

After Elizabeth's ordination, Bishop Epting asked her to start a new church in nearby Coralville. Knowing that Harper, with his MBA and organizational skills, would be Elizabeth's perfect partner, Epting asked him to co-found the New Song Episcopal Church, which opened its doors in 1994. For several years, Harper somehow managed to live his semi-secret gay life while working as a deacon, a professor, and a theater company director. He finally retired from the university in 2002 and from New Song Church in

2006. Yet during the week I spoke with him in July 2017, Harper had already performed a baptism and a funeral service and was still active doing pastoral work with hospital patients from the church.

As John got older, he began to get cranky, Elizabeth told me. "I don't think his vision has changed of what is valuable, what's good," she said. "But now I think he's more judgmental. (I think he would whack me for telling you this.) In particular there's little tolerance for Trump's implicitly racist presidency, and the fundamentalist Christianity that supports it."

Elizabeth's observation is consistent with what Harper tells me during our conversation: "I hope something will come along and quash conservative Christianity, which is one of the great enemies of everything I believe in." It puzzles him that Evangelical Christians have embraced Donald Trump as a kind of savior figure. The theologians who appeal to Harper—people such as Brian McLaren and Diana Butler Bass—argue that contemporary Christianity has its priorities backward. "When you walk into a church," Harper says, "the first thing people usually ask is: What do you believe? Do you believe the same stuff as we do? Can you subscribe to our creeds? What most churches want to know, in other words, is: *Are you like us?*"

Harper believes that this attitude is utterly irreconcilable with the essence of Christianity. "When Jesus found men along the Sea of Galilee and said, 'Follow me,'" Harper says, "there was no such thing as Christianity, let alone Christian Creeds. Jesus stressed belonging over belief. It's only at the very end of the line that Jesus asked, 'Who do you believe that I am?'"

It's late afternoon. Harper slows down; his voice softens. Stories of his zigzagging life bring images of four different people into my mind. I ask if he has any regrets.

"I would say my principal regret is that over a long period of time I spent so much of my life, in my profession and in organizational, charitable, and religious organizations," he says. "I decreed one year that I was cutting down and that I would no longer serve on more than ten boards at any given time." We both laugh.

"But I think what went by the wayside," Harper says more seriously, "was a personal or romantic life. I had a number of kind of short- and medium-term relationships. But I have to say in all honesty that I never invested in any one of them enough to keep them strong and meaningful."

Harper pauses.

"Beyond a certain age," he says, "you're always asked: What's the thread that connects your whole life?"

I first heard the ancient Greek legend "The Fall of Icarus" in my teens. As the story goes, a master craftsman Daedalus and his son Icarus are imprisoned in a labyrinth on the island of Crete. To escape from the labyrinth, Daedalus fashions two pairs of wings out of feathers and wax. Father and son strap on the wings and rise like birds above the island. "Keep a middle course over the water," warns Daedalus. "If you fly too high, the sun will melt your wings." Icarus soars exuberantly skyward. The wax on his wings melts. The feathers slip loose and flutter in mid-air. Icarus plunges to his death.

In my early 50s, I lived my own inversion of this legend. One Friday night in July 2000, my family and I drove from Houston to the Texas Hill Country for a long weekend. By noon on Saturday, the temperature had already reached 100 degrees. My 19-year-old son Jake hopped on his new mountain bike and set out on the labyrinthine roads and dirt paths of the old cattle ranch in Wimberley where we had bought 18 acres of land. Late that afternoon, Letha (my wife at the time), Emma, and I slipped into the Blanco River. We floated in the cool green water, savoring the maidenhair ferns and spring-fed waterfalls along the riverbanks. After a while, Jake rode his bike down to the river and dove in: a bronze young Icarus dripping with sweat.

Around 7 p.m., we toweled ourselves dry and headed up toward our van. "I've never been on your new bike," I said to Jake. "Why don't you let me ride it back to the lodge?"

"Okay," he said. "But watch out for that long steep hill." I walked the bike from the riverbank up onto Red Hawk Road, got on, and pedaled up a gentle rise. The hot black pavement began sloping downward. At first the slope was gentle. Then a hand-painted road sign screamed: SLOW! STEEP, WINDING ROAD!

I flew down the steepness, leaning first into a left turn, then quickly into a right. The next turn melted my wings. I slid off the pavement onto a dirt shoulder and slipped down a steep patch of brush. The back wheel hit something very hard, tossing me upward toward a handful of limestone boulders. I'm not sure what happened next. My glasses went sailing. My helmet split in half. I think I somersaulted in mid-air, landed with a thud on a flat limestone boulder, and slid downhill into a gravelly patch that dug long deep scratches into my upper back and arms.

I tried to get up but blacked out. I wiggled my toes and moved my legs and arms. *I'm alright*, I thought to myself. *Just banged up in my lower back.* Dazed, I turned toward the road and began waving.

Jake ran down to me and began to cry. He thought that I had broken my back or ruptured my kidneys. "Don't worry," I said. "I'm not dying." I looked around for his bike. It was 10 yards further downhill, the rim of the rear wheel bent into the shape of a "V." "Jake, I'm really sorry about your new bike."

"Fuck the bike," he said.

Jake pulled me 10 yards uphill and laid me on the floor of the van. By the time we got back to the lodge, a quart of sweat had poured off my skin. I thought I could wash up in the pool and relieve my aching back. Three times I tried to sit up; each time my head went black. The van became a family ambulance.

Lying on my back, I glanced up at the darkening sky as the electrical poles scrolled by on Farm Road 3237. An almost-full moon was rising. When a nurse opened the van door at the emergency entrance to the hospital in San Marcos, I couldn't sit up. I was lifted into a wheelchair. I remember the face-down view of the cement walkway, the electric eye that opened the glass doors, and the emergency room floor.

At the emergency room, I received a shot of Demerol in my left buttock. At approximately 2 a.m., having been X-rayed and CAT-scanned, I was told by the attending physician that no bones were broken. They released me the next day with mild prescriptions for pain relief and muscle relaxants. After 2 weeks of unrelenting pain and muscle spasms, I went to a Houston orthopedist, whose X-rays showed that my pelvis *was* broken—in three places.

For the next 2 months, I lay in bed with plenty of time to think and dream in my Vicodin haze. For some unknowable reason, I was spared paralysis or death—on a beautiful summer night with the sun going down and the moon rising and the cicadas calling. Like Icarus falling out of the sky—except that I am Daedalus and should have known better.

That summer night taught me many things. How easy it is to slip out of the world. How little it might take to die. Instead of blacking out and coming to, I could have blacked out and stayed out. Just gone from the world. I had always thought that Gabriel's trumpet would sound in all seven heavens when I die. Now I think it will be more like slipping quietly off the stage, leaving life's theater by the back door.

There is a deeper learning for me here: I inverted the ancient father–son story of Daedalus and Icarus. What happens if Daedalus flies too close to the sun and Icarus survives? In that case, Icarus is bereft of a father who might guide him to safety and prepare him to fly on his own.

My son was spared that fate, and I was granted another chance to get it right.

PART III | What Is the Meaning
of My Life?

| # Hugh Downs
*Television Broadcaster as Modern-Day Cicero*

Hugh Downs pulls up for our lunch in his shiny four-door white Mercedes. He has just returned from New York, where he celebrated the 60th anniversary of NBC's *The Today Show*, which he co-hosted with Barbara Walters from 1962 to 1971. Downs is an internationally-renowned television figure who began his career in 1949, the year I was born. In 1985, the *Guinness Book of World Records* awarded Downs the record for the most hours logged on a commercial television network—more than 10,000 hours. This was almost 15 years before he retired in 1999.

Downs wanted me to meet him at Don's Restaurant in the Hermosa Inn, built on the site of an old cattle ranch near his home in Paradise Valley, Arizona. He made a reservation there to ensure that we'd have a quiet place for lunch and a separate room for our interview afterward.

Handsome as ever, 91-year-old Downs walks up to me outside the inn, sporting a gray and purple patterned sport coat and white shirt sleeves held together by shiny nickel Indian cuff links. He shakes my hand firmly. I have recently read that the strength of a person's grip is a good predictor of longevity. I start wondering about my own grip.

We walk inside the Hermosa Inn and turn left beneath an arched, adobe-colored passageway into the restaurant. He sits down with his back to the window. Throughout a radio and television broadcasting career that spans more than 70 years, Downs maintained his persona as an affable and reassuring figure. His demeanor in person today is no different. I am, in effect, one of his viewers.

Downs was born in 1921 into a poor family in Akron, Ohio, where his father worked for a locomotive company. During the Great Depression of the 1930s, the family moved to a farm outside Akron and eked out a living. They raised chickens, kept a large vegetable garden, ate what they needed, and sold the rest at roadside stands. Downs absorbed a love of language and literature from his mother, who read aloud to him from Emerson, Dickens, Twain, and Tennyson. While working on the farm alongside his always curious and talkative father, Downs became fascinated with the universe—how it began, how it works, and what its workings mean for human nature and human life.

In 1938, Downs left the farm to attend nearby Bluffton College on a scholarship. While he was attending Wayne State College, to which he transferred from Bluffton, his father asked him to find a job in order to help feed the family—an unlikely prospect during the Depression. On a whim, Downs walked into a nearby building that housed the local radio station WLOK in Lima, Ohio and asked the receptionist what it took to be a radio announcer. The program director, as it turns out, had just lost his regular broadcaster and was looking for a cheap local announcer. He asked Downs to read an advertisement script and hired him on the spot. Thus began one of the great careers in radio and broadcast journalism of the 20th century.

After WLOK, Downs worked at various radio stations throughout the Midwest, finished his degree at Wayne State, and married his lifelong partner Ruth Shaheen. After a stint in the Army during World War II, Downs started his television career at NBC Studios in Chicago. Over the course of a dizzying career—he worked in a puppet show, a soap opera, a game show, and hosted *The Today Show*—Downs matured professionally at the same time television emerged as a mass medium. He developed a signature persona as a calm, thoughtful, and reassuring television presence. Downs' smooth and affable demeanor secured his place as one of the most trusted news people in American television.

When we began, I had no idea that Downs was a polymath and adventurer whose career took him all over the world. In 1982, for example, he learned that scientists had determined more precisely the location of the earth's axis at the South Pole and were traveling to mark the new spot. Downs contacted the head of the National Science Foundation and asked to accompany the team to Antarctica. At 6:10 p.m. on December 10, 1982, he picked up the 15-foot bamboo pole that marks the South Pole's precise location and planted it in the correct position.

After lunch, we walk into the next room and Downs settles into a low, deep-seated green leather chair. Talking as if he has known me for years, Downs moves quickly into a discussion of theoretical physics—not a topic I was expecting to discuss. He wants to tell me about the absurdity of anyone trying to discuss what came before the Big Bang, the scientific theory of the Creation story. "If matter and time and space were all created in that instant," he says, "then nothing came before it."

So far I am following him. When he moves into the territory of quantum physics, I get lost.

"At one time we believed that the electron was a little tiny hard particle that had an electric charge out from it," he says. "It was going out by the inverse square law, so the farther out it was, the weaker it was—you know?"

I don't know.

"Then we found out it wasn't a little tiny hard ball," he continues, paraphrasing Einstein,

It wasn't anything but a locust, and it was the electric charge that was the electron. But then we found the electric charge was a warp in a space–time continuum, and the warp was pure geometry. Pure geometry is pure math. Pure math is pure thought, and we are created in God's image, because we think. . . . Isn't that a neat idea?

He grins. "Because we *think.*"

Downs loves to think. He is curious to the core, which is a wonderful trait to behold—except that his thinking is difficult for me to follow. For Downs, God means different things at once. Sometimes he speaks of God as a metaphor for transcendent mysteries, as the uncreated Creator, as the One who conceived, thought, and created the world as if it were a clock that operates according to natural laws that scientists can discover. Quantum physics, today's version of natural law, leads straight to the mind of God.

Honestly, I can write these words but I do not fully grasp them. Ancient philosophy I can follow. Contemporary physics I cannot. How physics helps us understand aging I can't see until later in the conversation.

Talking quantum physics, Downs is in his comfort zone—a worldview honed over a lifetime that offers him an intellectually clear and personally satisfying explanation of the universe, including aging and death. I wonder: What should I say next? Should I admit that I don't quite grasp his point and ask him to elaborate? Or should I move on, since I really want to know what he thinks about old age and what his everyday life is like?

I shift gears.

"What do you love?" I ask.

"Ah, I love music of many kinds. I love the study of physics. I love the physics of music." For Downs, the love of music and the love of physics come from the same source: the purity and elegance of their highest forms.

As Downs speaks of his love of music, I begin to follow him. For 10 years, he hosted the PBS musical broadcasts *Live at Lincoln Center*. One evening, when he was interviewing the great cellist YoYo Ma, Ma said to him, "I hear you are a composer. If you write something for the cello, I'll play it." Downs had played violin and piano in his youth and began teaching himself to compose in his teens. He started the cello piece at age 72 and finished it at 80. YoYo Ma actually did premier Downs's cello concerto with the St. Louis Symphony Orchestra.

In his 90s, Downs says, his musical horizons have actually expanded, and he can hear intricacies of classical music that he never heard before. He talks at length about Beethoven's Ninth Symphony, completed in 1824 when Beethoven was stone deaf and could not hear a single note when it premiered in Vienna. After listening to every version of Beethoven's Ninth, Downs got the orchestral score and began studying what musicologists, conductors, and scholars had to say: "I found out that the first movement of the Ninth is terrifying. . . . [It makes you feel] the misery of life."

I have listened to Beethoven's Ninth Symphony since I was a young boy in the 1950s, playing vinyl records on the old single-speaker Zenith phonograph in the basement of our house. I too have felt the dark, bleak, and scary feelings arising from that movement, as it evoked the fear and disorientation that I felt—and still sometimes feel—after my father's death.

"What are the qualities of the music in the first movement that evoke suffering and fear?" I ask him.

"It's pure music," he says.

Here again was an appeal to purity—something untarnished, transcendent, leaving behind the impurities of ordinary composers and ordinary life.

A few years ago, on the last day of the Boston Symphony's summer season, I attended a performance of Beethoven's Ninth. I was in tears through most of the concert. I have always loved the fourth and final movement, the choral sections that transcend the suffering and fear of the first movement. The words of the choral music are based on Schiller's "Ode to Joy," a poem that celebrates brotherhood, friendship, and nature:

Do you sense the Creator, world?
Seek Him above the canopy of the stars!
Brothers—beyond the canopy of the Stars
Surely a loving Father dwells.

My tears are the closest thing I know to God—the emotional experience of being swept up by a benevolent force beyond my thinking self. The music is a prayer filled with love. It is thrilling, expansive, hopeful.

I don't think Downs yearns for God. I think he finds God in the purity of the highest forms of music and the most advanced forms of physics. The Greeks considered music to be a branch of physics; they showed us that harmony arises out of numerical ratios of sound waves. Instruments and voices produce sound wave vibrations that we hear as music—music that bursts into beauty and then fades silently into the universe. Listening to Downs makes me think about the beauty of aging, the beauty of each of us bursting into life and fading away after our lives have run their course.

When I ask Downs to talk about his own experience of deep old age, he talks about masculinity, particularly the challenge of reconciling manhood with physical decline. "Are you less of a man now than you were 30 years ago?"

"Well, it depends on what category you want to say," Downs replies. "Sexually, I'm much less of a man. Athletically, I'm much less of a man. Intellectually, I think I'm more of a man than I was then, in what I pursue and what I enjoy and take pleasure from." At the same time, he believes that he is more accepting of being old than he was in his 60s:

> It bothered me when—I bet I was not quite 60—when somebody wanted to help me out of a car. I was offended. Why would they think I needed help? It doesn't bother me now that people think of me as old, because I am, and it is comfortable for me.

Throughout his career, Downs has challenged ageism and our culture's dominant story of aging as decline. On the PBS program *Over Easy*, which won an Emmy in 1981, Downs launched his critique of ageism by emphasizing the uniqueness and value of all individuals, regardless of age. In 1979, when he was a mere child of 58, Downs published *Thirty Dirty Lies About Old*, an important popular book challenging pervasive negative stereotypes about aging and old people. Some of these "lies" include "Old age is an illness," "Old people have no interest in sex," "Intelligence declines with age," "You can't do anything about getting old," and "Older people stand little chance in a country that accents youth." Downs characterized these "lies" as sometimes conscious and sometimes unconscious, sometimes well-meaning and sometimes vicious.

"If we hang around long enough," he tells me, "loose lies will victimize all of us." In the end, Downs argues, it is a mistake to think that we have an aging problem. "Instead," he declares, "let's concern ourselves with individuals." It is a message perfectly suited to his television programs based on interviews with individual musicians.

In 1994, in a book titled *Fifty to Forever,* Downs revisited the problem of ageism in our culture and found little to be encouraged about. In particular, he worried that elders still found obstacles to exercising their rights in nursing homes and hospitals, including the right to privacy, the right to refuse treatment, "and ultimately even the right to die." In that book, Downs also acknowledged the growing potential for conflict between the rights and needs of older people and those of younger generations in an aging society. Still, in his steady, optimistic way, he saw "an improving picture. . . . The only obstacles are myth, injustice, and prejudice. And I believe we can remove them."

Downs's daily routine includes breakfast, morning emails, and 45 minutes of lifting weights, stretching, and riding a stationary bike—all while listening to classical music. "I like to keep what muscles I've got in good shape," he says. And right away he moves the conversation back to philosophy and physics.

"Even if your condition is perfect," he says,

> you will be overtaken by senescence. That is the second law of thermodynamics. If you can't live with that you're going to be an unhappy person. But if you can, you realize that it is a beautiful thing that young people get older and that old people get older. That is nature.

The second law of thermodynamics, Downs explains, is the immutable physical reality that all things—including human bodies—tend to a state of dissipation and dissolution before their elements are rearranged as new things. Downs understands physics not as abstract theory but, rather, as universal truth that applies to him as well as to everyone else. He is a happy person, partly by temperament and partly by living his belief that one who understands the truth of things will be wise and happy.

That doesn't mean aging has been easy for him. Along the way to his 90s, Downs underwent lumbar and cervical spine surgery, knee replacement, two kinds of eye surgery, and hospitalizations for serious systemic infections.

"What are you afraid of? Are you afraid of the future? Are you afraid of death?" I ask, probing for things that might not be accounted for by his philosophical stance.

"No," he answers quickly. "You can't *be* dead. Do you realize that?"

I look at him quizzically.

"Subjective death does not exist. You might see me dead, and I might see you dead, but neither of us would be dead because dead is *to not be*, so systematically and logically there is no such thing as death."

I smile at him, not quite sure if he's serious. His is a point of logic: You can't *be* dead because "dead" is not a state of being. If you're dead, you are not *being*. This, I think, is an intellectual sleight of hand. It may be logically true. But we all know that when you're dead, you're dead.

Downs has a fear of performing badly in the last segment of his last television show. "The funny thing about dying," he says, "is that it's so damned theatrical. My big problem is that I will do a bad job—that I won't perform properly. I have stage fright." I hope that Downs dies well in the privacy of his own family, maintaining those unique qualities that brought order, clarity, and comfort to those of us who watched him on television for so many years.

Some of what Downs says to me was written in his *Letter to a Great Grandson* on the occasion of his great-grandson Alexander's birth. The letter is a wonderful mix of autobiography, speculation on the stages of life (he lists 17 of them, lasting to age 110), and advice. Downs hopes that Alexander will read the 2003 *Letter* four different times in his life: as a boy, a young man, a middle-aged man, and an old man. "Nature is kind," he writes to Alexander. "At various times in your life you will not think so, but it's true." Speaking of his own multiple surgeries, infections, and hospitalizations throughout the years, Downs goes on:

> If I had known in advance of any of these impending miseries, I might have suffered some dread, but I didn't, and none of them was an ordeal. You will not escape troubles of this kind. But you will take them in stride, and your chances are good for as decent a life as I have been handed.

Downs's worldview is essentially that of the ancient Stoic philosophers, who believed that difficult experiences and negative emotions (e.g., fear, envy, or anger) could be overcome with knowledge and virtuous living. The more I listen to Downs, the more I am reminded of the ancient Roman statesman and orator Cicero. Like Downs, Cicero had little patience for those who resisted or opposed the order of Nature. "Enjoy the blessing of strength while you have it," he admonished his readers in *De Senectute*, "and do not bewail it when it is gone, unless, forsooth, you believe that youth must lament the loss of infancy, or early manhood the passing of youth."

At age 91, Downs may seem to have exceeded the limits of Nature's order. Actually, he is a contemporary exemplar of fulfilling Nature's possibilities.

He is a beneficiary of the dramatic increase in what gerontologists call *longevity*—the average age at death. We now know that human beings are built to live a maximum of approximately 120 years, what scientists call the human *lifespan*. This is something that Downs learned in his study of gerontology at Hunter College in New York. What we don't know is how closely our culture's increasing longevity will approach the human lifespan. Although recent data show regional disparities and decline in longevity among the poor, some scientists are predicting that the average age at death will continue to grow, even approaching 100 years.

Will most men (and women, who live on average 7 years longer than men) eventually live to 100 or 120? If so, will they be overstaying their welcome? There are those who think it would be best for all concerned if we only lived to an average age of 75. On the other hand, there are scientists who are working hard to cure the "disease" of aging and find biomedical interventions that will extend the lifespan—to 140 or 200 years or beyond.

I am someone who believes in living not "four score and ten" but five score. I am *not* with those who strive to extend the lifespan. I think: Let each generation have its day and make way for the next, as fruit falls from a tree. In Shakespeare's words, "From hour to hour we ripe and ripe. From hour to hour we rot and rot. And thereby hangs a tale."

In truth, Shakespeare's metaphor is difficult to translate into today's world of mass longevity, anti-aging medicine, and the biomedical quest to defeat aging. The problem is that we no longer know how long a generation lasts, how long our "tale" will be, how much burden we will be to society and our children, or even whether we can leave an ecologically sustainable world for those who come after us. Pursuing individual lives of greater and greater longevity is part of an economy and culture devoted to endless growth. Although Downs, like most of us, is hungry for more life, he also knows that endless growth is literally a dead end for humanity. Hence, he advises his great-grandson (and the rest of us) to live a life devoted to others, to promote an economy of service rather than growth. He believes, and I agree with him, that human beings cannot continue to treat Nature as mere material for our exploitation, extracting more and more resources from the earth's crust and polluting the environment with the waste of a carbon-based economy. That form of growth, he says, is "doomed."

After 3 hours of talking, Hugh Downs is getting tired. I reach down, grasp his hand, and help pull him out of the green leather chair to his feet.

I come away from my time with Downs in awe of his accomplishments (not least of which is his longevity), feeling unsure about my ability to fully grasp his ideas or convey his experience. But watching him pull away in his white Mercedes, I have that quiet sense of well-being and benevolence that emanates from his generous presence—an experience shared by millions of television viewers for more than 70 years.

Rabbi Sam Karff's biological clock wakes him up at 5:15 a.m. every morning, his favorite time of the day, when his mind is freshest sitting inside his dark, wood-paneled study. As the sun peeks over the horizon, Sam "davens," or prays, in Hebrew and in English—a ritual practice that renews his relationship with God and readies him for the day ahead: *Modeh ani lefanecha, melech chay vekayam. Shehechazarta bi, nishmati, bechemla raba emunatcha.*

"I am grateful to you, living, enduring Sovereign for restoring my soul to me in compassion. You are faithful beyond measure."

To this formal daily prayer Sam adds three personal concerns—what he's grateful for, what he needs help with, and what he hopes for. Sam's personal prayers these days center around Joan, his wife of 53 years. He oscillates between gratitude for their life together, hope for her recovery from ovarian cancer, and fear of losing her.

"Spare me from arrogance or self-denigration," he continues, "or from the notion that somehow I am diminished by the achievements of others. And God help me to feel more deeply the joy and pain of others, and help me to feel my own pain and joy."

I first met Sam in 1991 when I moved to Houston and joined his congregation, Temple Beth Israel, which he served for almost 25 years. Sam was in his late 50s then. He was President of the Central Conference of American Rabbis, served as the spiritual leader of 2,000 families, and regularly flew around the country speaking to Jewish and non-Jewish audiences. After he retired from Beth Israel in 1999, Sam worked half-time for The University of Texas Health Science Center at Houston, where he built a program called "Health and the Human Spirit," based on the primacy of meaning and connection in the doctor–patient relationship. Sam views medicine as a sacred (but not necessarily religious) vocation; for more than a decade, he taught medical students, interns, and residents about the humanistic aspects of health care, the essential difference between healing and curing, and the centrality of relationships in medicine.

In 2004, Sam foresaw the day when he'd retire from this second career and invited me to expand his program into a larger center. I would become his "boss," on the condition that I would let him know if he ever lost his mental acuity. (This never happened.) Despite some reservations, I accepted Sam's invitation and became the founding director of what is now the McGovern Center for Humanities and Ethics. Fear of letting Sam down was a primary motivation in the early years of my relentless drive to build the center during the next decade.

During the 25 years we've known each other, Sam has been my rabbi, my colleague, and my friend. Now he is somehow all three at once. So on this warm sunny afternoon, it is a bit awkward for me to interview him in my role as writer and scholar. We sit in his study, whose shelves are completely filled with books in Hebrew and in English. He wears a pair of light brown corduroy pants and a tan long-sleeved turtleneck shirt, his intense brown eyes gleaming beneath a strong forehead, his brown-spotted hands crossed gently across his waist.

When you talk with Sam, he rarely makes eye contact. Instead, he looks slightly above and to the left of your head. Maybe, I've often wondered, this is a way to avoid being overwhelmed by the pain of those who come to him for solace. Or perhaps he is afraid that you'll see into or through him to some darkness or insufficiency. Whatever the motivation, Sam's indirect gaze reduces your ability to engage him directly and limits emotional intimacy. It also allows him to formulate his thoughts unimpeded so that his brilliance and wisdom wash over you.

"You know, Sam," I say. "I have to ask you the same difficult questions I ask each old man for this book. And I have to write things about you that will not square with the way you see yourself."

"I wouldn't have it any other way," he says. "You call 'em the way you see them."

Sam (Schmuel in Hebrew) was born in 1931 into a family saturated with Jewish history, culture, and learning. His mother Rifka (Rebecca or Reba in English) was born in Jerusalem before World War I, when Palestine was still part of the Ottoman Empire. His father Eliezer (Anglicized as Louis) was born in the Russian Ukraine into a prosperous family of grain merchants who had migrated to the new city of Tel Aviv, at once seeking to build a safe Jewish homeland and fleeing from the constant threat of violent anti-Semitism. On his mother's side of the family, Sam is directly descended from Rabbinic royalty—in particular, Rabbi Israel ben Eliezer, later known as the Baal Shem Tov (Master of the Good Name), founder of "Hasidism," the 18th-century movement of Jewish spiritual revival in Eastern Europe. Sam is also directly descended from Rabbi Pinchas of Koretz, a leading disciple of the Baal Shem. It seems that Sam was almost genetically created for the rabbinate. His memoir is titled *For This You Were Created*.

Sam's parents married in Israel in 1922 and migrated to America for what they had intended to be a short interlude. They stayed for a lifetime. In the North Philadelphia row house where Sam lived with his parents and sister Elana, modern Hebrew was a spoken language. Like almost all first-born Jewish American sons, he was deeply loved—"even doted upon," he says. He was also expected to become a successful American man who exceeded his immigrant parents' accomplishments in education and income. Sam more than fulfilled these expectations.

And yet he lived—like all of us in one way or another—in a family where dark experiences at home left their mark on his psyche. As he notes in his memoir, Sam's parents often fought bitterly and relied on him, even as an 11-year-old boy, to mediate their disputes. Reba was a woman of great beauty, energy, and curiosity. Louis was a sweet and gentle man who taught Hebrew to elementary and middle school children after they had already completed a long day in public school. Reba, who was bitterly unhappy in the marriage, never considered Louis her equal and often spewed out her scorn in Hebrew and English. Louis rarely answered in kind but retreated from the struggle, hoping that Sam would restrain Reba. These long and painful rows split Sam down the middle. He loved his mother but could never give her all his love due to her treatment of his father. He loved his father but harbored a lifelong fear of becoming like him—a "loser." Sam's brilliant adaptation was to become a master mediator, a skill he used with great success in congregational and public life. The other, perhaps more important, response was finding his lifelong mate, Joan, with whom he shared almost 55 years of love and mutual respect and created a home, a refuge free of bickering, where they raised their daughters Rachel, Amy, and Liz.

On Saturday afternoons, when Sam was 11 years old, he traveled by bus and trolley to the Hebrew scholar Dr. Halachmi's home, where they studied *Sefer Ha-Aggadah*, later translated into English as *The Book of Legends*. This collection of rabbinic stories and folktales is a treasure trove of history, wit, and often cryptic insight that today occupies a special place in every rabbi's library. Unlike *Halacha*, the rabbinic body of legal writings that rule on behavior, the *Aggadah* uses stories, parables, fragments, quips, and sheer imagination to mine Torah for Jewish meanings, values, and religious truths that remain beyond the reach of the rational mind.

Those afternoons with this kind and learned teacher not only removed Sam from his family's toxic air but also grounded him in what at the time was a little-known tradition of rabbinic writing that opened his mind, heart, and imagination. The *Aggadah*, or Jewish Folk tradition, came to play a central role in Sam's theology and his style of congregational teaching, preaching, and lifelong study.

In 1949, the year I was born, Sam graduated from Central High School, a 1-mile walk from his home. That fall he entered Harvard University as a freshman, class of 1953. Although granted a full-tuition scholarship, Sam couldn't afford to live on the Harvard campus in Cambridge. For the first 2 years of college, he lived instead with his Uncle Abe and Aunt Scotta in suburban Newton. Like Sam's father Louis, Abe had also migrated from Tel Aviv to America. He completed law school and established a lucrative law firm in Boston, which allowed him to finance some of the extras, such as summer camp in the Poconos, that Sam and his sister Elana enjoyed.

Sam graduated from Harvard in 1953 at the height of "the American century," the era of unchallenged American military and economic dominance when our culture trusted in science, rationality, and unfettered progress. Harvard represented the pinnacle of masculine academic excellence and social prestige. Sam's experience at Harvard didn't fit the dominant image of Protestant masculinity that George Vaillant spent a lifetime studying. Like Catholics, Jews were under subtle pressure to tamp down their religious identity and loyalty. Harvard was their ticket to secular success. Sam's professors rarely expressed personal interest in religion. They studied it. Even Harvard Divinity School was reputed to be the place where students went to decide whether or not they believed in God. Despite Harvard's secularism, Sam's Jewish education and identity were expanded and nurtured at Hillel, the Jewish fellowship group on campus, led by Rabbi Maurice Zigmond.

By the time he had finished his rabbinical training, Sam came to the view that the key to faith lies not in religious doctrine but, rather, in stories— especially the stories that tie individual lives to Biblical texts. "I love to tell stories," he says. "I love to tell stories to children." The most well-known Biblical story, of course, is the story of the exodus from Egypt, when God parted the waters of the Red Sea to guide the Israelite people from slavery to freedom. Jews are commanded to tell this story every spring at the Passover seder and expected to link it to the struggle for freedom everywhere, including the oppressive darkness often hidden in their own hearts.

To help children see a connection between the Exodus story and their own lives, Sam often told a rabbinic tale about a man named Nachshon. As the Israelites flee from Pharaoh's army, they reach the swirling waters at the edge of the Red Sea. Moses orders the people to cross, but no one moves. Moses asks God to save His people. God waits. Finally, Nachshon plunges into the water by himself. At first the water comes up to his knees, then to his waist, then his shoulders. Nachshon keeps walking. Just as he begins to disappear beneath the waves, God parts the waters and the Israelites cross to the other side. When Pharaoh's army pursues the Israelites into the seabed, the waters come pouring back and all the soldiers are drowned.

"What is the meaning of this story?" Sam would ask his Sunday school classes. "Why did God wait to part the waters?"

Or, more provocatively, he might ask: "Would God have saved the Israelites if Nachshon hadn't stepped in over his head?"

Sam often used this rabbinic tale to help children understand that God expects us to move forward into the unknown, to be active in achieving our own freedom, redemption, or salvation. As my mother used to say, "God helps those who help themselves."

The story of Nachshon illustrates key elements of Sam's religious world-view: God has chosen to be self-limited so that human beings may have the dignity of free will. Although God loves his people unconditionally and forgives their sins, God demands moral accountability. This too derives from a sacred story. Soon after the Israelites cross the Red Sea, Moses climbs Mount Sinai and receives the Ten Commandments from God, inscribed on a set of stone tablets. When he comes down the mountain, Moses sees the unruly Israelites worshipping a golden calf. Enraged, he throws the tablets to the ground and shatters them. Only after pleading with God does Moses receive the second set that have come down to us.

Wonderful preacher that he was and still is, Sam's sermons seamlessly linked the stories of individual congregants to rabbinic stories, Biblical passages, and current events. He has the most remarkable spoken voice I have ever heard. Whether in the pulpit, at the lectern, or in conversation, Sam's voice is comforting and compassionate: It has an instructive quality that conveys a lifetime of learning without pedantry. I think Sam's voice also contains a subtle anxiety that seems to seek refuge in listeners' attention, admiration, or love. Thousands of students, parents, patients, clergy, and synagogue staff have happily supplied all three.

For five decades, Sam has poured out a deep and abundant body of sermons, essays, books, and lectures, often given on celebratory or difficult occasions—such as the talks he gave at the 350th anniversary of Harvard; the sermon he preached at Houston's Christ Church Cathedral after the terrorist attacks on September 11, 2001; or the invocation he gave at the second inauguration of George W. Bush. The sun streams through the windows in Sam's study. It is time to steer the conversation toward more personal yet universal topics—age, sex, and death.

"What is it like to be an old man?" I ask with some trepidation.

"I *am* an old man," he says, "and I bear the name honorably. I don't pussyfoot and say seasoned citizen or senior citizen. And I'm very grateful to be an old man who is still functioning as well as I am." Every morning, after prayers and a cup of coffee, while watching "Morning Joe" on MSNBC, Sam walks on a treadmill for 20 minutes and then lifts weights. Unlike Sherwin Nuland, who worked out at a gym and felt young, Sam accepts the challenge of adapting to and being compassionate toward his declining body. "It served you well," he says. "It's seen you through the other days, the salad days, and now be kind to it."

Sam regards old age, disease, and mortality as the price of being human. He takes the view of the great medieval rabbi and philosopher Moses Maimonides: Disease, old age, and death are not punishment for original sin, as they are for Maimonides' contemporary St. Thomas Aquinas. They are simply, Sam says in his book *Permission to Believe*, "the price we pay for being flesh and blood human beings who live in a natural world. We can feel enormous pleasure and intense pain. Suffering is the price we pay for the blessings of creation."

For several years, Sam and I walked a 3-mile loop in Memorial Park in Houston on Sunday mornings. As he got older, he had to stop more frequently. Then we reduced the distance to a mile or so. More recently, we've stopped walking and switched our Sunday morning time to eat breakfast together. A few years ago, a neuropathy in Sam's right foot made it difficult to distinguish the gas pedal from the brake pedal. After he barely missed hitting a young girl crossing the road in front of him, Sam voluntarily stopped driving. Many men would have denied this impairment and kept driving until their car keys were taken away.

Sam views old age and death as taxes. "We owe God a death," as he puts it. When I ask him about his own death, Sam begins by discussing the meaning of his life. "I've had a great life," he says, and if I die today, I would not feel cheated. I want to live, but I would not feel cheated. The source of meaning in my life comes from giving love and being loved. And I feel needed and useful, amazingly so. My faith is robust enough that my ultimate source of meaning—apart from love and being needed and useful—is the sense of Covenant with the ultimate One and a personal God.

Without arrogance or certainty, Sam believes that he has met the ethical demands of the covenant.

"Are you afraid of death?" I ask.

"I'm not afraid of death. I'm not afraid of death," he says. "I really feel that I'm not afraid of death because I've lived my life reasonably well."

Like most men to whom I talked, Sam fears "losing my grip mentally or being in a position where I'm tested and can't acquit myself honorably. I hope I am able to die before that happens."

By far Sam's most challenging experience as he's gotten older has been Joan's long struggle with ovarian cancer. I remember the day he first told me that she'd been diagnosed. We were sitting at lunch in a little bistro cafeteria below Methodist Hospital. I started to tear up but stopped myself because I wondered whether my tears would detract from the emotional support he needed. He was still working at the McGovern Center then, and we saw each other every day. I began calling almost every evening to find out how they were doing.

Interviewing him 3 years and one surgery after her diagnosis, I ask Sam if he could imagine life without her. He lowers his head and looks away. "I dread it. I dread it. Oh, I dread it," he says. "But I'll make the best of it."

Joan Karff, who died on September 2, 2016, was no retiring rabbi's wife. She was a formidable woman, to say the least. Although she read and critiqued Sam's sermons before he preached them and gave her full love and support throughout his demanding career, Joan was not a regular at religious services and maintained her own career as a dancer, choreographer, and volunteer program developer. For years, she ran "Women on the Way Up," a program in which she accepted a few minority high school girls each year and took them to the ballet, the Museum of Fine Arts, expensive restaurants, and discussed novels with them. When Joan turned 80, little more than a month before she died, 100 graduates of "Women on the Way Up" celebrated a reunion at the Karffs' home. Joan mustered the energy to appear with her usual grace. It was, Sam says, an immensely gratifying validation of her life, complete with a book about the program and coverage by a local television station.

Joan freely expressed opinions that were often politically to the left of Sam's views. On several occasions, I witnessed (or was subjected to) her powerful will, wit, and demanding intellect. Sam and Joan belonged to a monthly group of spiritually- minded friends that Thelma Jean and I have co-hosted for 10 years. One evening, I led the group in a silent, meditative exercise of simply listening to the sounds made by a Buddhist singing bowl and talking about the experience. Joan, who found these exercises useless, asked that we chose an explicitly political topic for discussion the following month. Since it was her turn to lead the next session, I suggested that she pick whatever topic she wanted us to discuss. "What about the refugees fleeing from Syria, North Africa, and the Middle East into Europe?" she asked, at least a year before the numbers rose from a few thousand to more than a million. "What does a country in Europe owe them? To welcome all refugees no matter what? To take them from the boats, feed and keep them safe until they can return?" With her uncanny knack for exploring uncomfortable issues, she led a powerful discussion the following month that anticipated the tragic and growing problem of people fleeing war, poverty, and drought, seeking a home in Europe or North America.

Joan's independence and forcefulness were often on display in more personal settings. At dinner with them, for example, you knew the evening was over when Joan picked up her purse and said, "OK honey, we're going." One afternoon, Sam and Joan were at the McGovern Center to attend a talk by Sam's friend Jeremy, a wheelchair-bound pediatrician suffering from brain cancer. As I wheeled Jeremy toward the conference room, I told him the story of Sam recruiting me to expand and direct his program at The University of Texas Medical School at Houston. "You'll become my boss," he had said.

I looked at Jeremy and laughed, "Sam Karff has no boss."

"Oh yes he does," said Joan who was walking along beside us.

Sam is not one to show his feelings, at least in public. Many of our Sunday breakfasts when he was talking about Joan's long and awful struggle with cancer, I would be the one in tears. Rarely, as if in response, he would tear up himself. He was so sad for so long. I watched his back bend more and more forward over those months, trying to carry the load of caring for her.

At the very end of her life, Joan was no longer able to get out of bed to go to the bathroom. This was an intolerable situation for her. Joan had been a dancer and directed a modern dance group in Houston for many years. Her body was a source of great pride. Losing control over it was hardly dignified. "Death with dignity," Sam said to me, "is mostly an oxymoron."

In August 2016, it became clear that Joan's death was imminent. She decided to allow Houston Hospice into her home. I had always felt close to Joan, and I was one of a small group of friends she would allow into her room to say goodbye. The day we had planned my visit, Joan took a turn for the worse and said we'd have to reschedule. Soon afterward, I left for vacation and never saw her again.

On Labor Day weekend 2 weeks later, my new wife Thelma Jean and I were in the Berkshires, staying in the 18th-century clapboard house on Fred Snow Road in Becket, Massachusetts, that we loved to rent every year. Early in the morning on September 2, my cell phone rang. It was Sam.

"Tom, Joan died at 3 a.m. this morning. I wanted to tell you."

I tried to keep from crying out loud. "I am so sorry. How did she go?"

I managed to ask Sam some questions about plans for the funeral, how he was doing, and said that we'd leave right away for the funeral. He said that we should stay for the rest of our vacation. "Are you kidding?" I said. He talked for a few minutes about the six decades they had together.

What I remember most is the last thing he told me: "Enjoy it while you can."

After Joan died, Sam lost his capacity to pray. Overwhelmed by grief, he couldn't get out of bed or remember the words of the early morning prayers. Gradually, he recovered this spiritual practice and added a new sentence to his davening: "Guard over, sustain the soul of my beloved Joan in eternity, in the world to come."

When I interviewed Sam again a few months after Joan's death, he acknowledged what we both knew. "Yeah, it's a difficult journey," he told me. "There's no doubt about it. But it's the life journey, and I've been blessed. I really have. I haven't been spared, but I've been blessed."

| James Forbes
*Old Man by the Riverside*

Reaching 392 feet into the New York City skyline, Riverside Church is one of the tallest churches in America. Its front entrance looks out at Grant's Tomb along the Hudson River. From the rear entrance, you can walk across Claremont Avenue to Union Theological Seminary or down the street to Columbia University. Perhaps the most famous church in America, this imposing neo-Gothic structure was built in 1930 with money donated by John D. Rockefeller, Jr. For almost 60 years, Riverside was the nation's premier bastion of liberal Protestantism. Its "whiteness" wasn't apparent until 1989, when an African American from the South—Reverend Dr. James Forbes, Jr.—was installed as the fifth Senior Minister. He served in that capacity until his retirement in 2007 and returned again in early 2014 as Interim Senior Minister because Riverside's racially divided congregation still hadn't found a permanent replacement.

In March of that year, I fly to New York and take a taxi to the back entrance at the corner of 121st and Claremont. Inside a long hallway, a dozen homeless black men doze on benches lining the dark wooden walls. Light slips in through sooty stained glass windows. I take the elevator to the 19th floor and walk to Forbes' office, which is set behind a front room that houses his young white male assistant. Forbes is a strong, upright, and handsome man. His green, slightly watery eyes contain a complicated mixture of his life's experiences: love of preaching, a radiance alert to the Pentecostal realm of the Holy Spirit, and hurt and anger from a lifetime of experience with white racism. Dressed in a brown three-piece suit, Forbes is his usual dapper self.

At first the interview is awkward. Trying to help Forbes remember me, I mention that my wife Thelma Jean is the beautiful woman in his congregation who waits in line to talk to him at the end of Sunday services. I remind him that we are friends of Walter and June Wink and that I had interviewed Walter for this book when he was in the latter stages of Lewy body dementia. I also mention my old and deep friend Connie Royster, a development officer at Yale Divinity School whose phone call convinced Forbes to see me. That seems to orient him.

I begin by asking about race at Riverside, a topic I'd long been wanting to talk with him about. This is a difficult subject for Forbes because he wants to protect Riverside's reputation and still acknowledge the very real and painful racial problems that have plagued him here. On the surface, it seems strange that a church devoted to universal rights and diversity would founder on the rocks of racial division. But, as a book on Riverside's history puts it, it is one thing to have a "Negro in the narthex" and quite another to have a "black preacher in the pulpit." Under his predecessor, the powerful, white, Presbyterian activist William Sloane Coffin, African Americans made up 38% of the congregation. Under Forbes, that figure rose to 60–70%. As soon as he arrived at Riverside, more blacks began filling the pews, the men in suits and women in their Sunday best or wearing colorful tribal robes and turbans. Gospel, jazz, spirituals, and reggae resounded inside Riverside's lofty walls. Forbes' Pentecostal past moved into Riverside's present.

Born in a segregated area of Raleigh, North Carolina in 1935, Forbes was raised in a household swaddled by generations of preachers. As a child, he often stood on a coffee table and imitated his father's fiery preaching style. His mother worked as a maid for a white family across town and then came home every day and cooked dinner for her family of 10. Every night, Forbes remembers, she checked to see whether all of her eight children were present; if anyone was missing, the other children prepared a plate and put it in the oven in order to keep it warm for the missing sibling. As he notes in the book on Riverside's history, this ritual gave rise to an image of God as "mama eternal, who before I can eat asks, are all the children in?"

In the American South of Forbes' youth, blacks were not allowed to use "white" bathrooms, eat at "white" restaurants, stay in "white" hotels, or sit in the front sections of movie theaters or buses. Nor could they buy houses in "white" neighborhoods, where they could only get menial jobs working as domestic help, laborers, or postal delivery men. In their own communities, life revolved around the church, the place where blacks learned to develop their talents; compete with and look after each other; and hear, feel, and praise the spirit of God. Forbes spent much of his childhood in his father's Providence Holiness Church, a Pentecostal church whose intensely emotional style of preaching opened him to the Holy Spirit and to the importance of worship, serving others, and loving one's enemies.

From slavery to Jim Crow to the present epidemic of police brutality against black bodies, African American religion is infused with the struggle for freedom and the desire to move—one might say—from oppression to expression. It literally gives voice to the struggle and creative search for the full range of life's options.

In Forbes' tradition, the intensely emotional experience of the Holy Spirit frees preachers to perform inspired acts of God and deliver special messages of revelation. Preaching, dancing, swaying, singing, and call-and-response are vehicles for transcending the rules of racial domination and creating spaces for freedom of expression. These experiences were burned into Forbes' soul. "We 'Break into the Spirit,'" he says when I asked him about his Pentecostal preaching, and he begins to sing "O freedom, o freedom, o freedom over me."

Forbes has always been a great lover of all kinds of music. His call to the ministry came in an unorthodox way. One night, when he was still in college at Howard University, Forbes put on a recording of Tchaikovsky's Fourth Symphony and heard the voice of God:

Jim Forbes, don't you know I have called you? Don't you know I have called you?

When Forbes applied to Duke Divinity School, he was told that "Negroes" were not welcome. Despite his father's fear that his communion with the Holy Spirit would be destroyed by spiritually empty liberal intellectuals, Forbes attended Union Theological Seminary, where he studied with the theological giants Paul Tillich and Reinhold Niebuhr. In 1960—at the outset of the civil rights movement—he returned home to North Carolina to work at his father's church. Along with his brother David, Forbes took part in the first sit-in protests at the lunch counter at the Woolworth department store in Greensboro, where blacks were traditionally denied service.

After various preaching and academic appointments, Forbes went back to Union Theological Seminary, where he served as professor of preaching from 1976 to 1985. As he matured, Forbes grappled with his professional identity and his preacherly voice. One night, as he was returning home from Union, he sensed that there was someone behind him. It was Jesus. A soft, strong voice rang in his head. "You believe that to be a good Christian minister, you have to be a very unselfish person, almost selfless, and that you should serve other people," the voice said. "I need to let you know that I am not a person whose giving to others preempted my responsibility to care for myself. That is not who I am." From this encounter, Forbes says, he realized the importance of both giving *and* receiving, of caring for himself, and of having the audacity to be himself.

At Riverside, Forbes' ability to be himself was sorely tested. To some, his sermons were foreign—even alienating. Forbes' tradition is suspicious of any attempt to limit the work of the Holy Spirit through an overly scripted sermon or service. Except for his introductions and conclusions, Forbes always works from just a few handwritten notes. The direction and inspiration of his sermons come in the experience of preaching itself and are not bound by any prescribed clock time.

For all its genuine inclusiveness, Riverside was accustomed to a style of preaching and ritual that was "white." Its congregants, that is, were accustomed to the emotionally restrained, intellectual tradition that began with its first minister, Harry Emerson Fosdick. It was a tradition of advocacy for social justice, privileging the head over the heart and the mind over the body. Within 6 months of his arrival at Riverside, a faction in the church wanted to fire Forbes.

I witnessed some of this racial division firsthand. Toward the end of Forbes' tenure at Riverside—around 2006–2007—Thelma Jean and I often went to New York and attended Sunday morning services in that magnificent Gothic cathedral. We walked up from the subway stop at 116th street, entered through the back doors, and took the stone staircase that winds up into the sanctuary with its great vaulted ceilings, stained glass windows, uncomfortable wooden pews, and the quiet murmuring of gathering congregants. The sanctuary was designed to emphasize the greatness of God and the smallness of "man"—an effect accentuated by the sculpted stone pulpit that rises a good 15 feet above the floor and extends out slightly toward the congregation.

As a "preacher's kid," Thelma Jean was used to being near the action at the First Methodist Church in Dallas, where her father was Senior Minister from the mid-1940s to the mid-1970s. At Riverside, she also liked to sit up front, the better to see and be seen, by Forbes and the choir. I, on the other hand, was never comfortable sitting in the first few rows of a church or temple—as if I'd fail a quiz on the day's message or the clergy would see through efforts to conceal my lack of virtue. So we settled on 20 or so rows back on the pulpit side.

One Sunday morning, during a contentious period at Riverside, Forbes came down from the pulpit during the middle of a sermon. He was talking about reconciliation. As he walked through the congregation, Forbes approached certain people—black as well as white—offering to shake their hands and pray for their fellowship. Not everyone reached for his outstretched hand. Seemingly unfazed, Forbes walked back up to the pulpit, raised his voice to a fever pitch, and intensified his call for the congregation to open their hearts to God's love.

For the longest time, I admired and appreciated Forbes, but I couldn't connect with his preaching—its freewheeling, improvisational form and the escalating waves of emotion, physical movement, and occasional dancing and singing.

I grew up in a Reform Temple in New Haven, Connecticut, that was analogous to Riverside. Intense emotion was more or less banned. As a 16-year-old at my grandfather's funeral, I sat in the back as a pallbearer with the men in my family. When I broke down and sobbed, my grandmother looked back at me from the front row with a disapproving look on her face. At Temple Mishkan Israel, there was no notion of one's personal relationship with God. We listened to a choir hired to sing for us, accompanied by an organist who wasn't a member of the congregation. There was very little Hebrew and no give and take between cantor and congregation. There wasn't even a remnant of the fervent Eastern European musical tradition of the "hazzan"—a male cantor who praised and pleaded with God on behalf of his congregation and sang using ancient musical markings.

In the late 1980s, I felt the call of Jewish renewal and the need for a quickening of my own spirit. The word "God" came into my vocabulary, although I didn't (and still don't) have a fixed idea of who or what God is. In the early 1990s, I went to Philadelphia to meet Rabbi Zalman-Schacter Shalomi, a mystic and spiritual virtuoso like Forbes. I participated in a weekend "kallah," the Jewish equivalent of a revival meeting. Although Zalman's style of worship was somewhat foreign to me, I was drawn to him and excited to learn and absorb more spiritually charged practices.

As I thought about Forbes' spirituality and my own experience of Jewish renewal, I realized that I simply took a spiritual path, rooted in my own heritage. Eastern European Hasidism, translated into American culture in the 1990s, is simply a different spiritual idiom, a different way up the mountain. I believe that all paths meet at the summit.

But spirituality is not a belief. It is the emotional experience of being connected to God or to one's image of ultimate reality. As I sit in Forbes' office and listen to his plea for spiritual renewal as well as his struggles at Riverside, something in me opens. I feel more aware of my own emotional limitations, of a wall that protects me from feeling inadequate or unworthy of God's love. For a few moments, Forbes helps me feel lighter and more open to passionate religious connection. These feelings, usually confined to romantic love, lead directly to my next question for Forbes.

When I ask about the role of intimacy and sexuality in his life, Forbes offers a view unlike any of the old men to whom I spoke. It is strikingly free of any worry or concern with stereotypes of black male sexuality. His answer is roundabout, culminating in humor and deep insight achieved by playing off his congregation—in this case, me. "I think that the older you get," Forbes says, "the more sexuality becomes de-centered from—"

"Orgasm," I say, finishing his thought.

"Orgasm," he says.

"This is interesting," I say,

because when I talked to Paul Volcker and a few other guys, some of them say, "I can't do it anymore. So I don't feel like I'm as much of a man." But that's not your view. Your view is that the nature of sexuality changes.

"Yes, that's right," Forbes says,

However old you are, you discover that sexuality is important not only for release or relief. Much like a mechanic tunes up a car, sexuality can tune up a relationship. And my sense is that, whatever vitality remains, whatever form of sexual satisfaction you come to, it can remind a couple that their love is strong even if the orgasm isn't as strong.

Forbes, I think, is articulating a crucial point about sexuality in later life. He focuses on the erotic give-and-take between what each person needs and what the other can give. And he has disdain for sexual assistance from pharmaceuticals or physical devices. I ask what he thinks about men taking pills such as Viagra or Cialis to offset their declining ability to have an erection. "I'll tell you what I think about it," he says. "I'm glad you asked that question. I'm on a soapbox. Please put this in your book."

"Go for it," I say.

Forbes launches into an attack on the pharmaceutical industry and its exploitation of men's fear of failure. Old men ought to form a union, he laughs, organizing against the high-priced pills guaranteed to give men long-lasting erections.

"What do you say to a younger man who worries whether he'll be able to get it up?" I ask.

"I would say," he replies,

"that when the Psalmist in 139 says that 'I am fearfully and wonderfully made,' you should recognize that sexuality is an even more remarkable gift than you were aware of . . . sexuality covers such a wide range of possibilities that it can be as much a look without a touch. It can be a look that invites touch. And I would say that just as a person who is blind develops a keener hearing, so various sexual erogenous zones respond. When the genitalia are not functioning as they had, sex doesn't disappear. It just finds another way to provide communion of spirit that reaches out for bodily manifestation."

His Biblical answer surprises and inspires me. For Forbes, sex and spirituality are not split apart. They are united in love. By linking God's wondrous making of our bodies to sensuous pleasure, Forbes frees us from the cultural taboo against sex in old age. And by linking physical and spiritual communion, he undercuts the traditional, constricted, masculine view of sex as phallic penetration. "Wouldn't that be something," he says, "if each person respects the other's needs and gives as best as they are able? Wouldn't that be wonderful?"

"Do you remember when you challenged the congregation to recite the 139th psalm every day for a month?" I ask. Forbes nods. " 'It will change your life,' you said. We never did get through a whole month, but we especially love verses 7–10":

Wither shall I go from your Spirit? Or wither shall I flee from your presence?
If I ascend up into heaven, you are there: If I make my bed in the grave, behold, you are there.
If I take the wings of the morning and dwell in the uttermost parts of the sea:
Even there shall your hand lead me, and your right hand shall hold me.

"We're going to have those verses engraved on our tombstone," I say.

When I ask Forbes about death—whether he is afraid of dying or of death itself—his answers are as unconventional as they are about sex:

I used to answer that question to Betty, my wife, by saying, "If God has something for me to do on this earth, I believe God can keep me alive and healthy enough to do it. But when I've completed what I was supposed to do, why keep scrabbling so hard?"

He pauses and says, "So that's part of my answer. I do believe that there will be dread. I would hope that there would not be panic at the thought of dying."

"What happens next?" I ask.

"My thinking is that we do not know," he replies,

and that I appreciate the effort of biblical imagination to say we're going to walk the pearly gates and all of that. I do not have a well-illustrated map of what the Celestial City will be like. I think that death invites us to release the description to the force that is beyond us. Intimations from people who say they've had near-death experiences, fine. Be glad to enter the light they speak of. But I think we shouldn't be fundamentalists about death. I think we should be philosophers about death. And I think that we should be content with metaphors that speak of continuation without asking for the description of form.

In a fascinating way, Forbes combines the language of his father's church and the ideas of modern hermeneutics he learned at Union Theological Seminary. On Easter, he preaches the language of resurrection: "He lives, he lives!" But he thinks in terms of Jesus' continuing influence rather than Jesus' return to earth. And that is how he thinks of himself, his continuing influence on those who live after him.

After 18 years, Forbes decided that his work at Riverside was done, that it was time to find other venues for his work of spiritual renewal. "I was not ousted," he tells me. "I retired on my own terms. I left here on June 1, 2007."

"I remember the day clearly," I say.

That morning, the issue of race still stalked the sanctuary. There were two outside speakers in the pulpit: the African American scholar and radical public intellectual Cornel West and the well-known white television producer Bill Moyers, himself an ordained Baptist minister. Moyer's theme was simply: "Jim Forbes is my pastor." West took a different tack. At the conclusion of his remarks about finding a new Senior Minister, West—with his wild hair and graying beard—looked out over the congregation, pointed his finger like a prophet, and warned: "We'll be watching you."

Now, as we sit in his office, Forbes is serving in the less pressured position of Interim Minister. He isn't bitter. But he acknowledges his frustration and disappointment. "I don't think I was successful," he declares. "If you are preaching in a secular culture in a church that has a corporate mentality, then what is the process by which you help them to understand spirit?"

"My basic spirit is still a congenial, pleasant, reconciling approach to things," he continues,

> I do not have the pressure now and have been able to say from the pulpit, "Guess what? I'm here as your transitional minister. I'm not trying to develop forums of groupies. I don't need to get anybody to think well of me. I'm here to preach the word of God as best I see it, and I hope you'll dig it."

From the segregated South of his youth to the nominally integrated North of his ministry at Riverside, Forbes—like his father and his father before him—has struggled all his life with various forms and degrees of racism. I keep thinking of the song "Old Man River" from the 1927 musical *Showboat*, sung by a character who's "tired of living but scared of dying." I mention the song to Forbes. He instantly starts singing, and I join in during the refrain: "Old Man River, he don't say nothing. He just keeps rolling along."

"Anything come to mind?" I ask.

"Yes," he says. "Old Man River talks to me about love having the last word. The triumph of good is what I hear in that song."

Early one evening in the spring of 2006, I drove my car up to The Spires, a condominium complex near the Texas Medical Center, and told the security guard that I was visiting my colleague Dr. Goodrich. The guard waved me on. I took a deep breath, handed the valet my keys, walked past the front desk, rode the elevator to the 10th floor, and pushed the doorbell to apartment 1005. Thelma Jean opened the door with a smile and grace that split me wide open.

Not long before, some friends had given a dinner party and invited me along with Thelma Jean and several other friends. I sat down at the table, patted the chair seat next to me, and asked Thelma Jean to sit there. She was wearing a pink suede jacket that I will never forget. After dinner, while Leonard Cohen's song "Bird on a Wire" was playing in the background, I admitted that I didn't know either the song or the artist. The next week, Thelma Jean came by my office and handed me a copy of Cohen's latest album, *Ten New Songs*. Leonard Cohen, I discovered, is a melancholy soul whose lyrics take you into dark and frightening and confusing places. And then they surprise and redeem you.

Once inside Thelma Jean's apartment, I sat on the couch. She sat in a chair across from me. We were both faculty members at The University of Texas Medical School at Houston, where she directed the Behavioral Science program in Family Medicine. We talked about the importance of preserving the human side of medicine in a world dominated by science, technology, and commercial pressures. We came back to Leonard Cohen, especially to the breathtakingly beautiful refrain from his song "Anthem": "There is a crack in everything/that's how the light gets in."

Thelma Jean asked if I had heard the song "Love Calls You by Your Name."

"No," I said. "Will you play it for me?" She turned on an old cassette player:

You thought that it could never happen
To all the people you became
But here, right here
Once again, once again,
Love calls you by your name.

Neither of us had any conscious intention of romance that night. But self-deception is a powerful thing. Both of us were in long, loving relationships. When we met, we understood ourselves being drawn into deep connection based on shared interests in the role of stories in healing and educating medical students. This was true, but it was only half of the truth. Terrified and electrified, I kept wondering what I was doing there. At this point, any sane and reasonably happy man would have turned and run.

What was I doing? I was 57 years old, ensconced in a long marriage with two grown children. I was not unhappy. I wasn't looking for a new relationship, certainly not with a Southern woman 9 years older than I was, and a Methodist to boot. Why would I risk disrupting my life and hurting my wife and children? For what?

But I was no match for Leonard Cohen's lyrics:

I leave the lady meditating
On the very love which I, I do not wish to claim,
I journey down the hundred steps,
But the street is still the very same.

In the following weeks, I turned the situation over in my mind. In all my 30 years of marriage, I had never gone alone into the home of another woman. I left that night wrung out by tension between desire and fear. I had never slept around, as they say. I had often been attracted to other women but never broke the rules of monogamy.

I sought advice from dear friends, told them that I was torn between my marriage and a new love. "You've never followed your heart before," said my friend Marc Kaminsky.

"Who are you to turn away from a gift that God gives you?" my friend Rabbi Richard Address asked me.

Thelma Jean was also feeling a passion she hadn't planned on, something she couldn't say no to. We both felt drawn into a force field we couldn't understand. Neither of us staked a claim on the other. But each of us felt claimed.

"Remember Truman Capote's line," she said, "'You can't own someone, but someone can own you.'"

We kept our relationship a secret for months, thinking we could somehow live double lives. That was not the only thing we deceived ourselves about. Later that fall, I left my marriage and told my children about my relationship with Thelma Jean. They were devastated. A few months later, my daughter Emma, who was hurt and angry at me for years, asked if I was happy. "I'm the happiest I've ever been and the most miserable I've ever been," I said. "Why?" she asked. "Because of the pain I'm causing."

Saying yes to new love catapulted me into the most wonderful and painful and confusing life. It opened me to an intensity of feelings I had never felt before. I faced terrible guilt from the pain I was bringing into the lives of people I loved. It took years to rebuild my relationships with my children.

This love came to me unbidden—from where? God? Destiny? Is there any cliché I can find to describe it? Passion that grows inside yet comes from a place beyond is impossible to grasp. I suppose that's why we need poets like Leonard Cohen.

I didn't ever know how closed I was, how afraid of opening my heart wider, how much of my passion had been channeled into my work. But here it was: more love, more life. More delight, more fun, more joy laced with guilt and wrapped in passion.

Thelma Jean and I were married in 2008. Love called me by my name, and I answered.

PART IV | Am I Still Loved?

| # Dan Callahan

*Love in the (Old) Age of Ethics*

On a crisp clear December morning, I take an early train from Manhattan to Garrison, a lovely hour's ride up the east side of the Hudson River. Dan Callahan picks me up and we drive to The Hastings Center, the nation's first bioethics think tank that he co-founded in 1969. He is now 83 years old, President Emeritus of The Hastings Center, and working on an ambitious book about major public health threats throughout the world. We walk to his office, where he sits with his thin, blue-veined hands crossed across his lap, dressed in corduroy pants and a beige sweater with a long-sleeved black undershirt peeking out from his wrists and collar. His mind is clear as ever.

I've known Callahan since the 1980s, when he was in his 50s and one of the most prominent bioethicists in the country. In fact, he was one of the founders of bioethics, a field that sprung up in the 1960s when technological advances in medicine had provoked new moral questions in health care, biomedical research, and the life sciences. Callahan has spent much of his life asking difficult questions: What is a reasonably but not excessively long life? What is a tolerable death? How much should society spend on health care aimed at prolonging the life of older people? Now he is living his own questions.

Callahan is a prolific and highly intellectual man. "I really like thinking of things," he says when I ask what he loves. He writes for 4 or 5 hours in the morning, reads for the rest of the day, and then goes for a walk. As am I, Dan is interested in the meanings and purposes of old age, and he worries that longer and longer lives are becoming more costly and burdensome to society. When we first met, he gave me a copy of his book *The Tyranny of Survival* and inscribed it: "For Tom Cole, a kindred spirit."

In perhaps his most famous and controversial book, *Setting Limits: Medical Goals in an Aging Society*, Callahan proposed that after we have lived out most of life's possibilities and obligations (often in our late 70s and early 80s), death becomes more personally tolerable and society should limit expensive life-extending medical procedures. Health care resources for those in deep old age should be devoted to care rather than cure. Callahan's emphasis on promoting a just society rather than extending individual lives did not—and does not—play well in American culture and politics: His book enraged many people when it was published in 1987. But controversy is also good for sales. The book sold almost 80,000 copies and was a finalist for the Pulitzer Prize.

When I invited Callahan to Houston more than two decades later, he was 80 years old and still a firm believer in his theories. I asked him to lecture on his new book *Taming the Beloved Beast: Why Medical Technology Costs Are Destroying Our Health Care System*. Much to his delight, he alienated virtually everyone in the room by pursuing a series of provocative questions: Why invest millions and millions of dollars in highly expensive technology or drugs designed to prolong individual lives (usually old ones) by a few months? Why not rethink where our health care dollars go and prioritize public health, prenatal care, nutrition, and health promotion programs that will add more years to many more people's lives? How do we build a society that ensures justice between generations? These were not congenial questions for an audience of surgeons, oncologists, scientists, biomedical researchers, and hospital CEOs who have spent decades pushing the boundaries of biomedical technology and working to cure or prevent the leading causes of death: heart disease, chronic lung disease, accidents, cancer, and stroke.

Callahan was born in Washington, DC, in 1930 to Roman Catholic parents of English and Irish extraction. Although his father, Vincent F. Callahan, Jr., had only a high school education, he hustled his way into newspaper and radio journalism and later into the management of radio stations in New Orleans and Boston. Callahan doesn't say much about childhood or early family life in his autobiography *In Search of the Good*, but his mother Anita clearly bore the brunt of a chaotic situation. As he puts it, "She was too often left at home by an alcoholic husband whose greatest pleasure was playing poker with his male pals in a back room at the National Press Club." Vincent Callahan's drinking and aggressive behavior cost him more than one job and led him to belittle and intimidate his family at home. "I was always waiting for a put-down," writes Callahan.

Educated at parochial schools by nuns who were "a tough-minded bunch," Callahan was not an especially good student. In high school, he began to take religion more seriously and became a competitive swimmer, a pursuit that led to his acceptance at Yale University. Although his father and high school teachers feared he would lose his faith there, Callahan was actually inspired by his fellow religionist William F. Buckley, Jr.: "We Catholics were mainly interested in how he crashed through the Protestant culture barrier; one of our own had made it."

As a Catholic, Callahan was a curiosity among academics and especially philosophers who were overwhelmingly secular. Accepted into Harvard University's graduate program in philosophy, Callahan studied with professors uninterested in religion, politics, or history. His mentors stood in the contemporary British analytic tradition rooted not in experience or ethical choices but, rather, in logic, language, and evidence. They argued that (1) the only meaningful ideas were those subject to scientific verification, and (2) "facts" and "values" lived in different intellectual foxholes with no possible tunnel between them. These were precisely the ideas that Callahan challenged by inventing "bioethics," a field that required practical thinking about how to connect medicine and morality, scientific facts and human values.

Even while he was at Harvard, Callahan was active in the world of lay Catholic magazines and liberal intellectuals, a world he shared with Sidney deShazo, who married him in 1954 and graduated, as she says, "magna cum baby" from Bryn Mawr in 1955. They were ardent Democrats and devoted followers of Dorothy Day, the leader of the Catholic worker movement who exemplified a life devoted to others without concern for one's own material well-being or security. This fervent Catholic ideal, writes Callahan in his autobiography, "meant accepting all of the children God sent."

Between 1955 and 1965, Sidney gave birth to seven children, one of whom died in his crib after only 42 days. In the next 20 years, Sidney emerged as a prominent "pro-life" feminist in national debates on abortion. During that same period, Dan fell away from Catholicism, dropped his opposition to abortion, co-founded the Hastings Center, and raised the fresh flag of bioethics over the moribund territory of moral philosophy in medicine.

As Callahan lost interest not only in Catholicism but also in questions of God and faith per se, his interest in secular morality grew stronger. Friends urged him to find a university post to feed his family. But Callahan found university life boring and lifeless, and he never made his living inside the walls of the university. "I knew I wanted to be some kind of philosopher but not in a university and not doing theoretical ethics," he writes in his autobiography. And so, at age 39 with a family of six children, Callahan hatched the idea of an ethics research center. In 1969, with psychiatrist and friend

Willard Gaylin as co-founder, he launched the Institute of Society, Ethics, and the Life Sciences, informally known as The Hastings Center.

After lunch in The Hastings Center's seminar room, we walk back to Callahan's office to pick up the thread of our conversation. He much prefers intellectual questions to personal ones, but I persist. "I can learn what you think by reading your work," I say, "but I can only learn about your feelings and experience as an old man by asking you about them." Callahan, it turns out, has been trying to learn the same thing about other old men by reading the biographies or autobiographies of Winston Churchill, Franklin Roosevelt, Trotsky, Machiavelli, Bernard Berenson, and Ben Bradley of the *Washington Post*. "I'm particularly interested to see what happens at the end of their life," he says, "and, of course, they all die. That's interesting too."

When Callahan imagines his own death, his greatest fear is asphyxiation. "So many older people say Alzheimer's is their fear," he says. "No, no. Having been in breathing crises, I will take Alzheimer's any day." Callahan sleeps with oxygen at night. His lungs are plagued by life-threatening emphysema, asthma, and allergies. I wonder how his current health affects his daily routine, especially his relationship with Sidney, and I ask about the role of intimacy and sexuality in his life.

"Basically disappeared," he says,

Partly because I can't "get it up" anymore, as they say. It's interesting: There are some things in old age that you once loved but that you don't have or miss anymore. I don't have sex. My wife and I haven't had sex in eight or nine years.

"Do you think that makes you less of a man?" I ask.

"No. Never," he laughs. "I guess I think more of myself as an old person." His voice trails off. "I don't know . . . old man . . . I don't know."

The question of masculinity clearly isn't one he's given much thought to. Nor is it a topic that interests him. On the other hand, his wife Sidney—an accomplished scholar and author in her own right—has written much throughout the years about being a woman. "Do you think she thinks of herself as an old woman or as an old person?" I ask. He suggests that I find out for myself. After a quick phone call to Sidney, we walk to the car and drive approximately 40 minutes to their home in Garrison.

Sidney Callahan is a beautiful woman. When we meet, her short gray hair is parted down the middle and curls below her ears. She wears a black turtleneck beneath her gray wool cardigan sweater, her fingers and wrists adorned with familial rings and bracelets. A Catholic woman of means, Sidney says that she was raised to value permanent things such as family, religion, art, and friendship. She points to two rings she wears daily—her mother's and her stepmother's. "All these women who helped me, I carry around with me all the time," she says. "I always say behind every man is a woman. Behind every woman is another woman."

Throughout her long life, Sidney has produced thoughtful, engaging, and serious work that springs from a deep Catholic faith. She has given countless lectures and workshops throughout the country, received eight honorary degrees, and authored or edited 13 books on parenting, family life, moral decision-making, suffering and spirituality, and abortion. Whereas Dan is on the pro-choice side of the abortion debate (they edited a book on abortion together in 1984), she represents a kind of "conservative feminism" in which the fetus "as sacred life" trumps any appeal to the mother's desire or life circumstance. Despite her conservative pro-life position, she holds progressive social and political views, and she remains open to theological positions outside of a rigid orthodoxy. She writes in a warm, patient, and generous voice.

From her upbeat tone, it might appear that Sydney is naturally joyful, patient, and loving. But her spiritual and intellectual accomplishments are hard-won. Her parents were divorced before she can remember. She was led to believe that her mother was dead, but at age 9 she found out that her mother had actually been hospitalized for schizophrenia, which led to her own fears about mental illness. "I'm a person who knew early in life that things were bad and you just seek the goodness," Sidney says. "I think that's why I am a religious person."

I'm thrilled that Sidney agrees to talk with me. There is a marked difference between interviewing a man by himself and talking with his wife as well. As with almost all the men in this book, Dan depends for his well-being on the love, support, and health of his wife. Yet he also works in the tradition of white, male, heterosexual philosophers whose writings have little or nothing to say about the role of love and relationships in their lives.

As soon as I sit down in their living room, Sidney cuts to the chase. "I'll tell you one thing—and forgive me for this," she says. "But I'll ask Dan a personal question and he'll give me an intellectual answer."

When I ask about sex, she says that it's no longer important:

> If it doesn't matter to Dan, it's not going to matter to me. So I came to terms with that. The great thing about having only one love and one marriage and one sexual experience in your whole life is that you never have any comparisons, and there's never any option or thought about anyone else.

I ask Sydney what it's like to be an older woman. "Women face all the issues of aging much, much earlier," she says. "That's why they age better when they really get old."

Three years later, I return to talk with the Callahans again. Sidney is 83, Dan 86. It is a cold, rainy December morning. Fog hangs over the Hudson River. When Dan picks me up at the Garrison station from the 10:45 a.m. train, I barely recognize him. He is gaunt. The curls in his hair have given way to stray wisps of gray. Within the past 6 months, he's been hospitalized three times, once almost dying of appendicitis. When we get out of the car in his driveway about a mile from the station, Dan steadies himself. Barely shuffling one foot in front of the other, he leads me up an outdoor set of stairs, through the back door, and into the kitchen of their modest two-story house. As we sit in the living room, their densely decorated Christmas tree huddles against the wall, working hard to convey the joy of the season.

I have returned not only to talk to Dan about his life at 86 but also to get a fuller picture of Sidney and her perceptions of Dan. What is it like to be married to him for all these years? What is it like now? What is her experience of being an old woman? First I speak with Sydney alone for an hour, then with Dan alone, and, after lunch, with the two of them together. The conversations are moving and sad and inspiring.

"What's life like every day with Dan?" I ask Sidney.

"Well, it's bad. It's hard because he is so unhappy and he's suffering," she says. "So my job is to take care of him—to keep his spirits up, be companionable, try to bring as much stimulation in as possible, try not to sink down into his sinking. You know?"

Sidney is particularly worried about Dan because he's closed himself off from potential sources of help—especially psychoanalysis, psychology, or meditation—that would require him to delve deeply into his psyche. Dan, she thinks, lacks the spiritual and psychological resources to find meaning or comfort in the midst of physical decline, a problem not uncommon among old men.

"I think it would be horrible to be an old man in this culture—terrible, terrible," Sidney says. Her ironic point is that because women have already lived without control over their lives or their bodies, they have already learned to make the kinds of adjustments needed to live well in old age.

Sidney is of course talking about herself and women of her generation and social class. "You've always had to deal with male privilege." (She estimates that she's cooked 25,000 meals during her lifetime.) She continues,

And if you've been pregnant, which I have been seven times, you know what it's like to be physically limited and totally unable to do this or that, and you have to become dependent and interdependent. Women are trained at interdependence, and that's what I think is a great advantage.

Sidney's health is still holding up well, although she is going blind and worries about the time when she'll be unable to read. Although she doesn't have the energy of youth or middle age, Sidney manages the household, goes to yoga classes, and visits with friends. Their son Stephen lives upstairs, checks in on them, and does whatever heavy lifting needs to be done. Sidney and Dan don't need more help yet. They are on the threshold of the Fourth Age.

After an hour talking with Sidney, a voice rings out from the other room, and then:

"Hello!"
"Hello?" says Sidney.
"Are you all watching the time?" Dan asks.

It's my cue.

In Dan's study, the shelves are still packed with resources needed to write his most recent book, *The Five Horsemen of the Modern World: Climate Change, Food, Water, Disease, and Obesity*. But after 47 books and more than 450 articles, Dan no longer has energy or desire for what has always been the inevitable next project. Parkinson's disease, emphysema, asthma, allergies, recent hospitalizations for pneumonia, and an appendectomy are taking their toll. It requires all his energy simply to go to the kitchen and unload the dishwasher.

"My daily experience of being an old man," he says, "is that it's basically a drag. And it's a problem, and it's getting worse, and it's not going to get any better, and I have to learn to cope with it." The main problem, he says, is that he's lost his desire to write. "If I don't write, what am I supposed to do?" he asks. "What do I do with the rest of my life?"

It pains me to see Dan so depressed. Were I in his shoes, I would turn to my family, my religious communities, prayer and meditation, and to whatever psychiatric help I could find. Yet I greatly admire Dan for his integrity. He is living according to his lifelong ideals, without flinching from the unhappy consequences for himself.

Dan is now confronting precisely the questions that he posed in the 1980s: What is a reasonably but not excessively long life? What is a tolerable death? In *Setting Limits*, he had put it as follows: A man has lived out a natural lifespan when "1) one's life possibilities have on the whole been accomplished; 2) one's moral obligations to those for whom one has had responsibility have been discharged; and 3) one's death will not seem to others an offense to sense or sensibility." Dan has fulfilled all the criteria of his own theory. He has lived a long-enough life, or what he would call a natural lifespan. But he is alive and unhappy. He doesn't believe in assisted suicide. "So this is really now *my* problem," he says. "It's hard as hell to know how long you're going to live these days."

"But do you still want to live?" I ask.

"Let's put it this way," he says,

> I still want to live but I don't care if I die. Now, the only thing is the impact on Sidney—she would miss me. I have no doubt she would survive quite well. But for myself, I don't care. I've done all I want to do. If I could get back into my old interests, I'd write another article on aging. But what would be the big deal?

In my own view, the quality of a long-but-not-too-long life is inseparable from the quality of love and connection we have to our closest relatives, lovers, friends, and local communities. However famous or accomplished, it is our primary relationships that make and sustain us—or they unmake and fail us. Dan's theory, I think, misses this point. It's why I want to probe Dan and Sydney's lives together.

After a lunch of some wraps, veggies, and brownies, the three of us move to the living room. Dan and Sidney sit on the couch across from me, and I set the recorder down on a table and tilt the microphone toward them.

Sidney is open about the joys and the difficulties that came with hitching her wagon to Dan's star. According to her, Dan promised that after he finished graduate school (he received his PhD from Harvard in 1965), it would be Sidney's turn to go to graduate school. Things didn't work out that way. Dan was consumed with founding and running The Hastings Center. There was very little money and six children. Sidney remembers that Dan had said no when she wanted to go back to school, even though he had promised to support her. Not one to be deterred, Sidney secretly squirreled money away for her education and finally received her PhD at the City University of New York in 1980 at age 47. Her dissertation was titled "Self-Consciousness and Promises."

"It's all about Dan," Sidney allows herself to say. "First it was about getting him through graduate school. Then it was starting his Center. Then it was

about his career. Then it was his books. And now it's all about Dan again."
She laughs as if to shrug it all off.

"I think at some point I did fail you," Dan admits,

I think you carry a little resentment to this day that I wasn't as helpful when
you wanted to make your own career as I should have been, partly because that
was coming exactly at the time I was starting The Hastings Center and working
round the clock to keep it going. What could I have done different?

"Kept your promise," Sidney says.

As I listen to them talk openly about their life of more than 60 years together, I see their complex mix of devotion and competition—devotion by
far the prime mover. Finally, I move to the issue that I want to pose to them.

"Tell me about the love you have for each other, what it means now, and
what it *has* meant," I say.

Sidney sighs. "You asked the wrong people because"—she pauses—"if Dan
were not here, I would give you a gushy, wonderful exposition about love."

At first, Dan is mute on this topic. I push him: "Is there anything left to
say about your relationship and its importance for the life you live now?"
Sidney's eyes meet mine.

"I don't know. I can't think of much," he says. After a long pause with his
arms crossed, Dan says a bit sheepishly in a low voice: "I'm lucky to be married to somebody so nice for so long."

Sidney laughs and makes kissing sounds. "Wow!" she says. "Thank you!"

"Say that again. I didn't hear it," I tease him.

"Don't make him. Don't make him say it again," Sidney laughs.

"I don't think those words made it into the recorder," I joke. "You're lucky
to be married—"

"To such a great person for so long."

| # The Story of Walter Wink

*Nonviolent Resistance and Dementia*

It is a beautiful sunny day outside Walter and June Wink's house, which is nestled alongside Route 8 in the Berkshire foothills of Sandisfield, Massachusetts. Snow lies on the ground around their country home, its whiteness broken by dead leaves and old wooden poles standing like crosses in the kitchen garden. Sitting across from Walter in his study, I lean forward and look at him in his flannel shirt, blue jeans, and sneakers, the contours of his long and still-rugged face marked off by wispy white hair and wire-rimmed glasses.

Walter is a prominent theologian, radical critic of the church, and peace activist from Dallas, Texas. At age 76, he seems already to have spent more than one lifetime of pastoring, writing, teaching, speaking, protesting, and loving. In recent years, though, he has struggled with restless leg syndrome (RLS), prostate cancer, and pneumonia. Now dementia, exacerbated by medication for RLS, is taking his mind and his life in terrifying pieces. Ever since he was diagnosed 5 years earlier, Walter has worked hard on all kinds of physical exercises and dietary regimens, neurological exercises, biofeedback programs, and treatments designed to slow or even reverse the progression of his dementia. But the dementia is a steady slide.

Sitting in Walter's study, we are surrounded by a lifetime of learning and by files for future books that will never be written and lectures that will never be given. Not sure where to begin, I look nervously past him at Buck Creek, water sliding over its banks and under a growing patch of ice. I am afraid that the interview will amount to nothing, and I am afraid of the despair in his quiet and hesitant voice. I am not sure how I will handle a conversation sure to be filled with confusing locutions, memory gaps, and moments of absence. I worry about the darkness and anger and confusion that will enter me. I have done many book and film interviews, and I know that people don't trust you unless you are calm and your heart is wide open. But then you can't control what comes in. You have to take it all. Perhaps I am afraid that his dementia will become mine.

We both comment on the strong gusts of wind outside Walter's study window. A sentence from John 3:8 comes to mind: "The wind blows where it wishes, and you hear the sound of it, but do not know where it comes from and where it is going; so it is with everyone who is born of the Spirit."

"Let me start with this question for you," I say, "and it's not an easy question. How different are you from the self you were 10 years ago?"

"Well, I was told by friends that the . . .," Walter hesitates and his voice gets weaker, ". . . that the experts . . . that the odds are very genuine and that you probably will be dead at some point in the next number of . . . There is one line probably . . . preliminary . . ." He stops in frustration and says, finally, "I can't do it."

We keep going, but our conversation is disjointed. Sometimes I can't get what he is trying to say. Sometimes there is nothing to get. Walter drifts between the present and the past, between presence and absence. He can't finish most of his thoughts or stories. I try to bring him back gently. Sometimes he is funny, and sometimes he is sad or resigned or vacant. I ask if he thinks much about God and wait through a minute of silence. "So where did your mind go?" I ask. "What have you been thinking about while we haven't spoken." "I was just checking in with the process theologians [who see God as a verb not a noun] to see if they are still thinking in those terms," he laughs. "They all seem to be doing pretty well."

I ask Walter if he can tell me about his contributions to biblical scholarship or if he will let his books do the speaking for him. "I may have no choice in that," he says, laughing. "But if I do have a choice I would say it's the passage from the Sermon on the Mount: 'Walk the second mile.'"

Fumbling through multiple versions of the New Testament on his shelves, I eventually find Matthew 5:38–41. Walter reads it out loud:

> You have heard it said that, "An eye for an eye and a tooth for a tooth." But I say to you, Do not resist an evildoer. But if anyone strikes you on the right cheek, turn the other also; and if anyone wants to sue you and take your coat, give your cloak as well; and if anyone forces you to go one mile, go also the second mile.

Walter can't really explain his radical interpretation of this passage or why it is the grounding of his fundamental message of Christian nonviolent resistance to oppression. Later, I find the answer in Chapter 5 of his book *The Powers That Be*, in which Walter claims, contrary to conventional opinion, that Jesus never recommended that Christians become doormats. When Jesus says, "Do not resist an evildoer," he is not counseling acceptance, Walter writes. That would be "an invitation to bullies and spouse-beaters to wipe up the floor with their supine . . . victims."

In *The Powers That Be* and in *Jesus and Nonviolence*, Walter argues that the gospel actually teaches a third way that is neither submission nor assault but resistance without violence. The phrase "turn the other cheek" does not mean to submit but, rather, to show the one who has slapped you that "his attempts to shame you into servility have failed." According to Walter, the phrase "go the second mile" was a response to the Roman soldiers who commanded Jews to carry their heavy military equipment for a mile. It means do twice as much as you are asked. Outperform the command and they will have no way to criticize your disobedience. As he writes in *The Powers That Be*,

> Jesus . . . is helping an oppressed people find a way to protest and neutralize an onerous practice despised throughout the empire. He is not giving a non-political message of spiritual world transcendence. He is formulating a worldly spirituality in which the people at the bottom of society or under the thumb of imperial power learn to recover their humanity.

According to Walter, "Almost every sentence Jesus uttered was an indictment of the Domination System or the disclosure of an alternative to it."

Walter's reinterpretation of these passages from the Sermon on the Mount was part of his effort to identify and preach about the historical roots of non-violent resistance, found later in Gandhi's movement against colonial rule in India; the nonviolent phase of Mandela's struggle against apartheid in South Africa; King's movement against segregation in the American South; as well as movements in Czechoslovakia, Poland, and many other places. Having identified the biblical origins of nonviolent resistance, Walter wanted to enroll contemporary Christians in the struggle against oppression. He himself traveled widely, witnessing the fierce dictatorship of Augusto Pinochet in Chile, as well as the poverty and oppression in the barrios and *favelas* throughout Central and South America. He slipped illegally into South Africa, where he taught and supported nonviolence in the fight against apartheid. During and after these trips, Walter often felt physically ill. He was overwhelmed by despair, lost weight, and could sometimes barely function. What saved him was not Jesus as the guarantor of salvation but Jesus as a practitioner and teacher of nonviolent resistance to oppression—Jesus, who understood, lived under, and challenged the evils of the Domination System and came to know that "neither death, nor life, nor angels, nor principalities . . . nor powers . . . will be able to separate us from the love of God in Christ Jesus."

After he reads the passage from the Sermon on the Mount, I ask Walter what he cares most about now.

"Well, one thing is that I have three books that I'm trying to finish before I give it up."

"What are they?" I ask.

"One is a collection of . . ."

"Essays?"

Walter stops. He looks at me in silent frustration, tears filling his vacant blue eyes. "I don't think I can do this."

"You can't do it? It's hard to remember the books?"

"Yeah."

Walter's extensive biblical scholarship was carried out primarily in the 1970s and 1980s, and it was driven by more than desire for academic advancement. (He was denied tenure at Union Theological Seminary, but Union later gave him its highest academic award a year before he died.) In essence, Walter wanted to humanize Jesus as a way of helping people claim and fulfill their own humanity.

Walter's last book, *Just Jesus,* was published in 2014, 2 years after his death. It is a collection of autobiographical fragments—some written before his death, some reprinted from earlier work, and some written in June's voice—completed with the help of friends and editors. In one fragment, Walter describes what he can of his complex and changing relationship with God in the course of his dementia. He had always thought that life-threatening illness would turn him more powerfully to God. "In fact," he writes,

the deeper I slipped into the darkness, the less I cared about God. Prayer was out of the question. In my journal, I once scribbled: "If I have a soul, it's silent. I don't know what the point of this book is anymore. If God won't heal me, God can go hang."

Later, he writes,

I had felt so strongly that God had called me to help others find meaning in life, but now the best I could offer was to give whatever my leftover self could offer. I felt like I was letting God down when I didn't use the gifts given me. And so I was afraid that I was a fraud. . . . I had a hard time being aware of God.

When he had to cancel workshops and lectures, Walter fell into a deep depression. He thought about suicide. But when the maker of OxyContin (the opioid he was taking for RLS) was fined for failing to warn the public about the painkiller's side effects, including risk of addiction and death, his family took him off the drug and Walter made a discovery. "I had not turned my back on God," he said,

> I hadn't lost my faith. I was being poisoned to death. . . . I feel certain that I would have died if my family had not gotten me off the drug. . . . I hadn't lost my faith. It was stolen from me. It was a new form of unbelief: "chemical atheism."

"Besides finishing your books," I ask him, "what else matters to you?"

"I do have fun a lot. . . . Joking around. I can talk better in those times when I am connected with—when I'm feeling good about my feelings."

"So you like to have fun, and you have fun when you are feeling good. And when do you feel good?"

"Mornings," he says.

"So Walter," I move on, "who do you love?"

"June, my wife, and life. . . . And my kids and I have the most remarkable . . . I wouldn't have anything come between that, and I don't think it will."

June has been an integral part of Walter's life ever since they got together in New York in the 1980s, when she was a schoolteacher at Riverside Church and he was a theology professor at Auburn Theological Seminary. Now the two are more intertwined than ever: She plays an essential role in maintaining Walter's life, his identity, and his dignity, which will include easing and presiding over his death. It is grueling and hard loving work.

In *Just Jesus,* June remembers that one afternoon after a nap, Walter came out of his room confused. He went to shave but instead picked up a book.

"You're sad," June said to him. "What are you feeling?"

"I'm going to miss you so much," Walter told her. They talked about death and dying and who in their family was left.

"I may be the one who dies first," June said.

"Chances are a 100 to 1 that won't happen," Walter answered.

"I will be the lonesome one. You will be fine," she assured him.

Walter broke down and cried and cried. June asked him if he felt better, and he nodded.

In the spring of 2012, when they were both exhausted from the long years of resisting and accommodating his dementia, Walter told June that he wanted to "be with Jesus."

"I could see that he had chosen to die soon," wrote June in the Preface to *Just Jesus*, "so one night I made his urn. As a potter, I felt that there was something beyond my hands forming this vessel. I made it quickly and went to bed." Walter died 10 days later.

During the course of his dementia, Walter learned to sing the Blues. At first, he chanted Psalms or songs he put together. "But I tried too hard, and they got all tangled up with my perfectionism," he writes in *Just Jesus*. "My spiritual guide, Andy Canale, had me create the blues on the spot, with no art or craft to spoil the spontaneity of the songs." Walter learned to sing his own blues, knowing that they were traditional tools to fight against the forces of domination. "The slaves knew that. When there is no conceivable hope, singing the blues opens up a new and other reality. . . . It doesn't have to be pretty. It can be a single note."

Walter and June learned to sing Christmas carols as a form of relief from the terrors of the night. "Every time June would sing and chant, I experienced immediate relief. . . . Singing carols alleviates nightmares, circular dreams, and sleepwalking. I have learned to accept my depression and work with it. Often I need lots of help." Almost to the end, Walter understood that living his life fully with profound memory loss could be a way of fulfilling the task of becoming human. Learning to accept his limitations allowed him to become more resilient, even to find light in the black hole of dementia. Dependency and vulnerability became the occasion of affirming his humanity. As his friend Andy put it, Walter was being challenged to live his own exegesis.

After an hour, Walter is visibly tired, and we move to the kitchen for a cup of coffee. When we come back, I return to the subject of faith.

"How important is your faith now that you are off OxyContin?" I ask.

"I've been a bit puzzled," he says,

When I have reflected on it, I don't feel like that. And I'm saying I'm surprised that I haven't done a lot of calling on God. I haven't been calling for help. On the other end, I have felt just fine. I accepted what God put on my plate. . . . And I figure I've had a terrific life, just beyond belief—with no expectations.

"What do you look forward to?"

"Good question. I don't know. I'm going to be dead pretty quick," he laughs. "That doesn't leave much . . . unless there really is life after death . . . leave much [he hesitates] . . . unless there really is life after death."

Walter falls silent. I ask if he remembers what he wanted to say. "Nope," he replies, it just—it's like we can't know and I'm happy. I don't need . . . I figure that if God is as good as people have been saying about him, there's a chance that there's going to be beautiful days on ahead. I wouldn't waste my time on an unnecessary expectation.

"If God is all he's cracked up to be, then you don't need to waste your time worrying about the afterlife. Is that what you mean?" I ask.

"Only if it's the opposite of the statement that God is so good he must— that he must be beyond belief," Walter answered. "Am I coming through? Are you understanding what I am saying?"

"I'm not sure," I say.

"Salvation's ultimate question," he says, drifting into profundity,

is that we have to save the planet. We have to literally save the planet. It can't just be a gesture. I mean total and absolute salvation, with everybody and every-thing. And that means doing the right thing ecologically . . . we need to expand the religious impulse . . . so that we can change fast enough to be salvific.

It is the end of our conversation. We are both tired. My face has been close to his for most of the 2 hours we spent together. What have I learned? I have learned that Walter's lifelong religious and political commitments still animate his much-diminished mind. These commitments are supported by caregiving relationships that hold and attend to his body, sustain his shifting identity, and maintain a dignity not otherwise available to one who can no longer control his body or his mind. Personally, I feel disoriented. I have opened myself to the intensity of Walter's thoughts and feelings and gestures that reverberate through me like a silver ball bouncing within a pinball machine, lights flashing and bells ringing until the ball inevitably disappears.

Sitting here in his study, I feel like the wedding guest who has just listened to the life story of the Ancient Mariner in Coleridge's famous poem:

He went like one that hath been stunned,
And is of sense forlorn:
A sadder and a wiser man,
He rose the morrow morn.

I look at Walter. His shoulders slump and his voice becomes even quieter. "I think I'm terrible . . . as somebody that's supposed to be helping people understand."

"You are the perfect, demented 77-year-old theologian of nonviolence and biblical exegesis," I tell him. "There's nobody else in the world that could do what you just did."

Walter laughs.

"Really. It's true. It's okay."

He laughs again.

"You think that's funny. Good. Good," I say. "Walter, you're the best. You're the best. Thank you."

"Okay," he says.

## CHAPTER 14

Ram Dass and Me

I'm sitting in my office in Houston staring at the computer screen. Suddenly, the Skype theme song pulses through the speaker. I click on the camera icon and there he is, zoomed in from Hawaii—gleaming green eyes, a big, slightly crooked smile, and wisps of white hair set off against the red–black quilt draped over the top of his chair.

"Ram Dass," I say, amazed that I'm actually seeing and talking to him. "How are you?"

"Just fine, just fine," he says, adjusting the camera until only his head is visible. Looking into his face, I take off my glasses and place my head between my hands, my elbows on the desk. My eyes brim with tears.

I've been waiting for this conversation for a long time, re-reading his books, viewing YouTube clips, watching the 2001 documentary *Ram Dass: Fierce Grace*. Before I interview someone, I try to absorb as much as I can and then face my inevitable fears. By the time we talk, I am ready for the encounter.

But this time my anxiety is stronger, the anticipation more intense. I know that Ram Dass is just another person. But another part of me believes that he possesses some sort of truth with a capital "T," some huge secret about the universe that will transform me.

At age 86, Ram Dass is a perfect screen onto which I can project my unspoken, half-understood needs and longings. He is his generation's last great American teacher of Eastern spirituality. In 1967 (the year I graduated from high school), he went to India as Richard Alpert, the Jewish Harvard psychologist. Transformed by an encounter with a Hindu guru, he returned as Ram Dass, "servant of god." He brought home with him an exotic tradition of Hindu yoga and meditation practices that eventually reached millions of spiritual seekers. His 1971 book *Be Here Now* has sold more than 2 million copies in English alone.

*Be Here Now* is part confession, part spiritual manifesto, and a completely original melding of Eastern traditions and Western needs. It appeared at a historical moment when Western religion had lost touch with its mystical traditions and practices of cultivating the inner life. Almost immediately, *Be Here Now* struck a chord with hundreds of thousands of people—not only those in the drug-saturated hippie movement but also young Americans who were looking for an alternative to the spiritual emptiness they felt in traditional religious institutions. Today, meditation, yoga, and other spiritual practices have become widespread. More and more people think of themselves as spiritual but not religious, eroding the membership and influence of mainstream churches. But in 1971, Eastern spirituality was considered strange and even dangerous.

In *Be Here Now*, as in the books that followed, Ram Dass tells his life story and outlines a plethora of Eastern ideas, practices, and resources for others in search of spiritual growth. "Now, though I am a beginner on the path," he writes,

> I have returned to the West to work out karma or unfulfilled commitment. Part of this commitment is to share what I have learned with those of you who are on a similar journey. Each of us finds his unique vehicle for sharing with others his bit of wisdom. For me, this story is but a vehicle for sharing with you the true message . . . the living faith in what is possible.

When I talk with Ram Dass, he is at the end rather than the beginning. But his message is the same. He talks to me about his long life with the honesty and vulnerability of a flawed holy man still seeking to work out his unfulfilled commitment.

By any ordinary standards, Ram Dass has fulfilled the commitments of many lifetimes. His interests range from environmental awareness and political action to international development—all seen through the lens of Eastern spirituality. His teachings are not sectarian. They are interlaced with Judeo-Christian sacred texts, stories, and images that yield what he considers universal or perennial wisdom. He has said that if Jewish mysticism had been alive and available in his formative years, he would not have turned to Eastern spirituality.

Before *Be Here Now*, Ram Dass wrote books as Richard Alpert on the topics of child rearing, LSD, and psychedelic experience. Since *Be Here Now*, he has written 11 books with collaborators. In addition to books and printed articles, his teachings are available in all possible forms: interviews, workshops and lectures, and documentary films (the most recent one released in 2017, titled *Going Home*). There are also countless web-based packages of his teachings on attachment, chanting, compassion, emotions, aging, dying, and death. Ram Dass' institutional and programmatic creativity is equally stunning.

In 1974, he established the nonprofit Hanuman Foundation, designed to embody the kind of spiritual service he absorbed from his guru. Out of the Hanuman Foundation emerged the Prison-Ashram Project, to foster the spiritual growth of prison inmates. With Stephen Levine, he conceived the Dying Project and later the Dying Center in Santa Fe, New Mexico, a residential facility aimed at supporting dying as a conscious process and as an opportunity for healing and spiritual awareness.

In 1997, at age 66, Ram Dass suffered a devastating stroke. Now, as I talk to him, he searches for words and for the power to speak. Early in our conversation, one pause lasts at least half a minute. He looks uncomfortable. I pull my chair forward.

"Do you need some water?" I ask, as if he is in the room and I can get it for him.

"No, I have it," he says, picking up a glass and drinking from it.

"I'm here if you need anything," his assistant Dassima whispers from behind.

At the beginning of our conversation, I can't tell if Ram Dass is looking at me. But if he is looking, he clearly sees my tears. I am embarrassed, but I know that compassion lives in his silence. I wipe my eyes, put my glasses back on, and gather myself. As the conversation goes on, he starts to feel like both an exalted wisdom figure and an old friend. He exudes joy.

"I doubt you'll remember me," I say. "We worked together in the conscious aging movement."

"In Florida," he smiles. Ram Dass does remember.

We first met in 1992, when we were teaching conscious aging workshops together in Florida and New York. It was the beginning of a movement devoted to helping people cultivate spiritual growth as they encountered the challenges of aging. Conscious aging was a way of resisting negative images of old people, saying "no" to the cultural story of aging as decline, encouraging people to live *with* the flow of time. Ram Dass was the leading figure along with Rabbi Zalman Schachter-Shalomi, whose book *From Age-ing to Sage-ing* later spawned a whole series of retreats and an organization that continues to flourish. Today, conscious aging is part of a much larger and varied cultural movement that goes by many names: positive aging, healthy aging, sacred aging, spiritual aging, and so on.

One morning in the spring of 1993, Ram Dass and I were sitting on the porch of a rustic building at the Omega Institute's Retreat Center in Rhinebeck, New York. I asked him what he thought about the soul. Was it immortal? Did it grow, develop, age, and die with the body? He wanted to know what *I* thought. "I think there is something immortal about us," I said. "But I don't know what it is, how to understand it, or how to experience it."

"Pure awareness has no age," he said. "It's like your mind waking up in the morning before it has a chance to think. Or a meditative state you reach when all mental clutter fades away and you are aware of nothing."

I laughed. "Why would I want to be aware of nothing? Then I could be ageless?" He grinned at me.

After Ram Dass' stroke in 1997, doctors said that he had only a 10% chance of survival. They underestimated him. "Three hospitals and hundreds of hours of rehabilitation later," he wrote in *Still Here* (2000), "I gradually eased into my new post-stroke life as someone in a wheelchair, partially paralyzed, requiring round-the-clock care and a degree of personal attention that made me uncomfortable." This experience taught Ram Dass that his previous spiritual teachings had failed to recognize that the body makes its own demands. Back then in his early 60s, feeling young and strong, he had naively viewed the body as merely a vehicle for the soul, something to be dismissed in search of the higher realm of the spirit. As he put it, "I ignored the body as much as possible and tried to spiritualize it away." The stroke plunged him directly into the Fourth Age, into a lifeworld of frailty and pain and dependency. It posed a severe challenge to his self-understanding and his spiritual practices—an issue that I wanted to explore with him in our Skype interview.

During the early moments of his stroke, when he was nearly dead and being wheeled down a hospital corridor, his mind went blank. "All I remember is the pipes, looking up at the ceiling," he recalled in the documentary *Fierce Grace* (2001). "Here I am, Mr. Spiritual, and . . . I . . . didn't orient towards the spirit. It showed me that I had some work to do, because I flunked the test."

Ram Dass' comments remind me of lying on my back in our white Chrysler minivan, being driven to the San Marcos hospital after my bike accident. There I was, looking up at the wires and telephone poles going by on those winding back country roads. Just looking up. Like Ram Dass looking at the pipes.

But is there really a "test"? What's wrong with just looking up at the pipes or at the telephone wires?

In Jewish mysticism, a righteous man aims to die with the word "Echod" on his lips. "Echod" means One in Hebrew. "The Lord Is One." Something like the Hindu goal of merging into the One by uttering the word "Ram" (God) as a person dies. When Mahatma Gandhi, leader of the movement for Indian independence from British rule, was gunned down leaving his house in 1948, tradition has it that he died with the word "Ram" on his lips. Perhaps this is what Ram Dass means by passing the test.

I admire these religious and spiritual aspirations. But they feel too lofty for me. I cannot reach them, and I do not want to be judged for failing. Now in my late 60s, I do not imagine my dying as a spiritual test. I do not aspire to die with the word "Echod" on my lips. I hope to die calmly, without fear and without pain, listening to my favorite music, being cared for by people who love me, having said goodbye to people I love, having tried and failed and tried again to live up to what the Talmud refers to as "The Ethics of the Fathers." I hope my children Emma and Jake will have forgiven me for the ways that I hurt them and will take the best of me on their own life journeys. I want my body cremated, and I hope that some deathless part of my soul returns to its Source.

Over the years and with great help, Ram Dass has turned a spiritual spotlight onto his physical frailty and turned it into his teaching. He continues to co-author books and articles. He Skypes into meetings. He remains Chairman of the Board of the Hanuman Foundation. Thanks to an army of actual and virtual assistants who promote his books, films, talks, podcasts, CDs, and tweets, Ram Dass is more visible than ever. If you Google "ramdass. org," you'll find innumerable ways to learn about him and his teachings. A quick trip to the webpage of his Love Serve Remember Foundation yields a stunning array of teachings, podcasts, events, features, and opportunities to buy popular products or donate. In 2017, the Ram Dass YouTube channel contained 771 videos, viewed by upwards of a million seekers. And the videos keep coming.

I do have to say that I am a bit skeptical of all this branding and marketing. Like the Wizard in the great 1939 movie *The Wizard of Oz*, Ram Dass communicates now by projecting an image of himself onto a screen— actually, onto hundreds of thousands of computer screens. In *The Wizard of Oz*, Dorothy and her friends pin their hopes on the "great and powerful" Wizard and set out on the yellow brick road to find him. After a long and arduous journey, they arrive in Oz. But when Dorothy's dog Toto pulls away the curtain that serves as the Wizard's screen, disappointed audiences see only an ordinary middle-aged man projecting a false self.

I wonder what I will find when I pull back the curtain around Ram Dass. I don't want to hear the stories and teachings that I've already heard and read over the years. I want to know what it feels like to be Ram Dass now. I want to get to know the man behind the great spiritual teacher projected onto digital screens throughout the world. Our encounter scrambles my thinking and changes me in ways I am still trying to understand.

Very slowly and very haltingly, Ram Dass talks to me about the tension between his spiritual aspirations and his own frail, everyday existence.

"My body tugs at my soul," he says. "I witness my pain. . . . I . . . identify with my soul but . . . my . . . pain . . . sometimes captures my . . . consciousness."

"What happens when you wake up in the morning?" I ask.

"Well . . . my attendants wake me up."

"Then what happens?"

"Oh boy . . . then toileting."

Ram Dass has severe nerve damage in his lower body. When attendants wake him up and transfer him from bed to wheelchair to toilet and back to wheelchair, Ram Dass groans and grimaces. They work hard to ease the pain in his back and legs and feet.

Dassima, who arranges his schedule, also handles physically intimate aspects of his care. "Every day . . . she takes a tube off my penis," he says.

"Then she has to clean up the urine and slip the tube back into your bladder?"

"Yeah."

"Every day?" I ask.

"Yeah."

"Oh shit, that's awful. No wonder you identify with your soul."

"That's right," Ram Dass laughs with me. "That's right."

After he is washed and dressed, Ram Dass sits in his chair and has breakfast—chicken soup. Then he plays with his cat and reads. (Naomi Levy's *Einstein and the Rabbi* is on his table.) Once or twice a week, attendants take him swimming in the ocean.

"So then maybe I Skype," he says, "for . . . conferences or lectures or . . . board meetings."

"Or you let people like me talk to you, which is very generous," I say.

He smiles. I feel the light of his countenance.

"I love your smile Ram Dass," I say, my voice rising. "It's the same smile. You have the same teeth. The same green eyes. . . . I mean, you really are *Still Here!*"

"YEAH!!" he says, almost jumping out of his wheelchair.

When he went to India in 1967, Ram Dass had no clear idea of what he was after. With his colleague Dr. Timothy Leary, he'd spent years experimenting with mind-altering psychedelic drugs that left him in the same disenchanted world where he had begun. In the secluded Kainchi ashram nestled in the Himalayan mountains, he met Neem Karoli Baba, the man who broke him open and became his lifelong guru, or spiritual teacher. Maharaj-ji, as Ram Dass calls him, was the man whose example and gift of unconditional love transformed Richard Alpert into Ram Dass. The second time he went to India, Maharaj-ji gave him the simple and impossible instruction to "love everybody and tell the truth." "I can't do that," he replied.

I don't know how to do that either. The instruction to "love everybody and tell the truth" has been Ram Dass' primary personal spiritual work or "sadhana." It is, for me, the equivalent of the Judeo-Christian instruction to "love your neighbor as yourself," or to love "the Lord your God with all your heart, with all your soul and with all your might." It is the spiritual work of a lifetime.

Neem Karoli Baba died in 1973. Yet he lives inside Ram Dass. "I dwell in my imagination," he says. "And my imagination is a room in my head or my heart. And my guru and I visit in that room."

Maharaj-ji is Ram Dass' guide to the next level of spiritual evolution, when the individual soul, the Atman, merges into Brahman, the cosmic soul, the eternal essence of the universe. Like the term Heaven in Christianity, Brahman is an impossibly vague yet essential aspiration toward a timeless realm that resolves all suffering. When Ram Dass meets with his guru, Maharaj-ji invites him to merge with him into Brahman.

"Can you do that?" I ask him.

"No."

"What's in the way?"

"I'm not ready to merge into the One. I'm in soul land," he answers, meaning that he still dwells in his individual soul.

"When will that happen?" I ask.

"Any moment."

"Well," I laugh out loud, "let me know when you are going. Put me in your suitcase. I want to come for the ride." He laughs along with me, but he is not joking. "Well," he says,

. . . any moment . . . . . . . . . . . . because my life is moments.
Moment . . . . . . Moment . . . . . . Moment . . . . . .
And these moments . . . they're not in time or in space. Moments are . . . . . . . . . . they're infinite. . . . . . . And you go, you delve . . . into the

moment . . . . . . the sun and the wind . . . . . . . . . and the people and the cat and the trees . . . . . . and the ocean. . . . . . . . . . . A moment . . . . . . all of that . . . . . . all of that. And you delve into that, you get into the . . . . . . One.

Inside these words and long pauses, I half-sense what he means. During one long silence, I have such a moment. I live inside it.

Once or twice a week, Ram Dass' attendants or friends take him down to the beach in an electric cart he calls the "Beach Bug." They swim, sing Hawaiian chants, and feel the joy of the sun and the sky and the wind and the clouds. One friend whom Ram Dass calls his "minister of fun" lives by the saying: "If it's not fun, don't do it. If you have to do it, make it fun."

"My life . . . is full of love and fun," he says. Love and fun intermingle closely with pain in Ram Dass' day-to-day experience. Like life and death.

"Ever think you've had enough?" I ask him.

"I . . . think about it every now and then."

From time to time, Ram Dass thinks about suicide, remembering the example of his friend the poet Stephen Levine, who killed himself when his brain began to falter.

"But that's up to Maharaj-ji," he says. "Maharaj-ji runs my life."

"I thought Dassima runs your life."

He laughs: "He runs her life."

I ask if I can talk to Dassima. She comes onto the screen.

"Ram Dass says that Maharaj-ji runs your life too."

"Yes, that is correct," she says.

"How? How does he do that? I don't get it," I say. "Maybe I'm not spiritually adept enough. I haven't gotten there yet."

Dassima laughs. "Well, he's just there."

Now it is my turn for a long pause, as it begins to sink in: Here is a gap I can never bridge with words or ideas. No matter how many questions I ask, I will not understand. Ram Dass and Dassima inhabit a different spiritual universe, a place of imagination and experience informed by a lifetime of specific commitments, community, spiritual practices, and teachings.

"Uh-huh," I say, responding to Dassima. "And when the time comes. . . . Ram Dass says when the time comes, he might just decide it's time for him to check out."

"At some point, it will be."

"Yeah, but how will you know? You take the cues from him, or will he take the cues from his guru, or both?"

"Well, I think what he meant was that when the time comes, he'll drop his body, and then his soul will soar."

I stop asking questions that beg for reasons and causes. I accept Dassima's spiritual metaphors: The body will "drop" and the soul will "soar." They point to a mystery beyond reason. Ram Dass envisions dying, even by suicide, as part of his spiritual evolution. But he is not ready yet. He is still working to erase the difference between himself and his teachings, between his experience and his screen appearances. When the two become one, Ram Dass will disappear.

It never occurred to me that so much of my own aging would be consumed caring for my mother, Jackie. In one sense, I have been taking care of her since I was 4 years old.

My mother was born in New Haven, Connecticut, in 1925. Like her father did, Jackie stands less than 5 feet tall and has never been prone to acknowledging or expressing difficult emotions. Like her mother Helen, she attended the prestigious women's school, Mount Holyoke College. After she graduated in 1947, her life's transformative milestones came in a rapid un-predictable sequence. In 1948, she married the love of her life, my father Burton Michel. In 1949, barely 9 months later, she gave birth to me. In 1952, she gave birth to my twin siblings, Patty and Paul. In 1953, Burton drove his car into a bridge and died a week later. In 1954, she remarried.

After my father died, my mother leaned on me. I felt her sadness, her de-pression, and her emotional absence long before I could name them. I tried everything to keep my mother from disappearing too. I tried to soothe her and to be the perfect little boy who could win her love. I tried to be the man of the house to protect my brother and sister.

But Jackie had problems I could never understand or control. She has al-ways suffered from depression and from some kind of personality disorder that splits her mind and her heart and leaves her with unpredictable bouts of rage and tears. My mother never could give me (or my brother and sister) the love I needed. She tried her best. And I kept trying to be perfect.

Barely a year after my father's death, my mother married Bertram Cole, who went by the nickname Bert, which sounded exactly like my father's nick-name Burt. When Bert Cole adopted us, my name was changed from Tommy Michel to Tommy Cole. I still remember my kindergarten teacher asking me if I liked my new name. My second father seemed to erase my first father. He became, simply, my father.

During my middle school years, my mother and new father began arguing and shouting at each other, waking us up at night when my mother would throw him out of the house. Sometimes she went through the phone book and asked me to call hotels to find out where he might have checked in for the night. Other times, I would run down the stairs and beg my father to stay, telling him how bad it would be if we were left alone with her. He would sigh, turn around, and sleep on the downstairs sofa.

In my high school and college years, my father, exasperated and exhausted, became bitter and domineering. Yet he still asked for help handling my mother. After I graduated from Yale University and moved a few miles from my parents in New Haven, he would ask me to come to the house and mediate fights, which, depending on the day, might include my mother throwing his clothes out the window or actually batting her own head against the wall. I refereed these fights as best I could. One Saturday morning, my father rode his bike over to my apartment, sat down, and burst into tears. I thought that he would never stop shaking.

If I hadn't left New Haven, I think my mother would have eaten me alive. I did leave in my mid-20s to pursue a PhD in American history at the University of Rochester. One holiday weekend when I was back in New Haven, my father and I went for a long walk around Lake Whitney and through East Rock Park. "It's a beautiful day, isn't it?" he asked in a far-away voice. And then: "I just don't know what to do with your mother. Nothing works—electric shock therapy, medication, psychotherapy."

By then, *I* was in therapy to save myself from being chewed up in the mad machinery of their marriage. Neither of them had any insight into their own inner world or ability to talk about their own experience.

"Listen," I said to him. "I can't do this. I am *not* going to talk to you about her anymore. But if you want, I *will* talk to you about how *you* are doing."

"That's cruel," he said. I looked away. After that, he bore the burdens of their troubles by himself.

In 2006, not long after they bought a house and moved to Venice, Florida, my father died at the age of 88. My mother was 81. The day after his funeral, my mother ordered that all of Bert's clothes be removed from the house. My brother, sister, and I dutifully carted them over to Goodwill. For several years after Bert's death, Jackie seemed happy. We dissolved a trust that my grandfather had set up to oversee her finances, allowing her to control the money she lived on. For the first time in her life, she was fully independent.

In her late 80s, my mother began to lose her grip. Checks bounced. Bills were misplaced and went unpaid. Bottles of Grey Goose vodka appeared more frequently in her recycling bin. Afraid for her safety, friends began putting her in a cab after they finished playing bridge. Soon she was dropped from the group. Jackie was at the beginning of both vascular dementia and alcohol dementia.

My mother has always lived by denial. She swerves unpredictably from sweetness to obstinance or rage if she doesn't get her way. After a long, agonizing process, my sister and I convinced her to move into an assisted living apartment at Ashton Gardens, where people could keep an eye on her and she could maintain a semblance of independence. The night before my sister and I planned the move, Jackie never went to sleep. She lay on top of her bed and never changed her clothes. She didn't even take off her sneakers.

"I am *not* moving. I changed my mind," she said in the morning.

My sister flew back to Atlanta later that afternoon. I stayed for the day, trying to figure out how to respect her diminishing autonomy while keeping her safe and deciding which of her affairs needed to be managed. That night, my mother got drunk and began shouting. "Get out of my house. And don't bother to call to see if I am alive or dead. . . . Treat me like a human being. For once in my life I'd like people to leave me alone."

When my sister called to check on things, Jackie switched bizarrely to a different channel on her personality radio.

"Oh, hi honey," she said sweetly. "Did you make it home safely? Yes, we're fine. Just having a quiet evening. I'll talk to you soon."

She hung up and returned to her rage.

"Who do you think you are? Mr. God? Mr. Yale man?" she said to me. "Leave me alone. You can't tell me what to do." I retreated to the guest bedroom and began writing in my journal. She spent the next hour muttering under her breath, puttering aimlessly around the kitchen, looking for things to put in order. Her own disorder could not be fixed.

In the next few years, I had to take over her finances, take away the keys to her car, and hire full-time home care. It was a painful and tumultuous period. She hated the arrangement. And it was terribly expensive. Sometimes my siblings and I agreed about what to do. Sometimes we disagreed angrily. In the late spring of 2017, we finally decided together to move her against her will into Tuscan Gardens residential care facility in Venice. It was a clever, stealthy, risky scheme, and we stayed out of the fray.

One morning, her caregivers took her to a doctor's appointment and then out to lunch. Meanwhile, movers came to the house, picked up her furniture and belongings, and set up the apartment we had rented at Tuscan Gardens.

She never went home. After lunch, the caregivers took her to her new residence. For a month, my mother was deemed a "flight risk" and needed tranquilizers and supervision. Then, to everyone's relief and astonishment, she calmed down and began enjoying the place.

Now, she eats in the general dining room and enjoys group exercises, games, and other social activities. Without access to alcohol, her mind is clearer and her mood better. It may be years before she will need to be moved to a locked "memory care" unit.

Caring for my mother is like having another job. I don't recommend applying for it, but if you are an aging child of an aged mother, the job will likely seek you out.

The job posting might look like this:

**Qualifications**
The successful candidate will
- Serve as Durable Power of Attorney
- Be of sound mind and body and reasonably competent in the midst of unreasonable circumstances

**Job description**

- Decide when and how much to intervene as your mother becomes compromised.
- Work with physicians and caregivers to devise safe and respectful systems of care.
- Combine respect and firmness.
- Become aware that you will revert to painful patterns of emotion from your childhood.
- Manage the fear and anxiety and the resentment provoked by your mother's rage, denial, confusion, and fluctuating competency.
- Confront your mother when checks start to bounce, bills get misplaced, and she spends hundreds of dollars monthly on payments to nonprofit solicitations.
- Learn to make decisions about finances, driving, household maintenance and repairs, competence, home health care, residential care, long-term care, and so on.
- Work with your siblings to create consensus about major decisions.
- Remember that your mother's well-being is primary and that the way you and your siblings care for her is the model your children will have when it becomes their turn to care for you.

A year after my mother has settled into Tuscan Gardens, I come to visit her for a weekend. I fly into the Tampa airport, pick up my rental car, and drive south on I-75 to Venice. We've just sold her house. Jackie has settled in well to her life in the residential care setting. She gets herself dressed every morning, goes down to breakfast, and spends the morning playing cards, attending exercise class, or getting her hair and nails done. When her mind deteriorates to a certain point, she'll move into a memory care unit on the other side of the common area. After years of conflict, I am relieved that she is happy there and that I'm not responsible for supervising her daily care and maintaining her house from 1,000 miles away.

On Saturday after breakfast, we drive up to Sarasota to spend some time at Selby Botanical Gardens, where there are more bromeliads and orchids than I've ever seen in my life. We walk along the path that opens out onto Sarasota Bay. She loves the view of the water and the Andy Warhol exhibit in the old Selby Mansion. As we drive back down Route 41 to Tuscan Gardens, she talks about losing her memory.

"It's terrible," she says. "I'm used to being independent. I can't drive. I don't have any money. I can't remember things. It's scary."

My mother has said these very words for years. I am tired of trying to reassure her.

"Yes," I say. "I'm sorry it's so hard for you."

"Look," she says in the next breath, pointing to the cloudless blue sky. "Isn't it gorgeous? Have you ever seen a sky like that? You can't improve on nature."

After we get back to Tuscan Gardens, I tell her that I'm going to take a nap for an hour at my hotel. "Why don't you just lie down in my bedroom? You can rest there."

"No," I say.

"Why? Just go lie down in my bedroom," she presses me.

"Just trust me," I say, needing a break. "I'll be back at 5 o'clock and we'll go out to eat."

At 5 o'clock, I pick her up, and we drive to an Italian restaurant in the strip mall on Jacaronda Boulevard. The service is slow. People at the next table are noisy. The long day is catching up with her. She stands up angrily. "This isn't working for me," she says. "Let's go."

"OK," I say. "Maybe we can find another place."

We drive around for 30 minutes. Long lines loop around every other restaurant in the area. "Let's go back to Tuscan Gardens," I say. "They serve dinner till 6:45."

When we get back, we can't find a table to ourselves in the dining room. We sit at the end of a long table, with one old man half-sleeping his way through dinner at the opposite end of the table. As soon as the waitress comes and shows us the menu, my mother shakes her head and gets up. She is wearing a faded blue-green blouse, her mouth slightly lopsided from the time she fell down drunk and had to get her teeth repaired. She glares at me through her still intense brown eyes. "I'm not eating this food," she says. "Take me back out. I want to go to another restaurant."

"No, mom, we're not going back out. We've already tried that."

In a flash, she comes out swinging. She orders me to leave. She pleads with me. Then she cries and shouts, "I can't believe you're treating me like this. I just want to go out for a decent dinner. Is that too much to ask?"

"Mom, we're not going anywhere. Just sit down and have something to eat. You're hungry."

The more I tell her that we're not going out again, the louder she gets. I speak to her calmly. I try being silent. I look away and eat my cold tasteless fish filet. She keeps giving me orders as if I am 4 years old. Her fury rises. She can't believe that I am actually refusing to do what I'm told. This goes on for 20 minutes. People around us are getting uncomfortable. Finally, I call the nurse on duty.

The nurse comes over and sits down. "What's the matter, hon? What's got you so upset?" My mother tells her a story that bears little resemblance to what's happened in the past 2 hours. The nurse's eyes meet mine. I ask if she can calm my mother down and take her back to her apartment. She nods. My mother is even more enraged. She turns to me and with a snake's venom in her voice, she says, "You've met your match."

*You've met your match.* The words reverberate in my head. In that moment, I finally understand: for her, it has always been a battle of wills.

I stand up and turn toward the door. The nurse promises to call me when my mother is safe in bed in her apartment.

"Bye, mom," I say.

CHAPTER 15 | Gleanings for the Path Ahead

My journey to meet the elders in this book was long and winding. Actually, it consisted of many journeys over a span of 6 years. It was an honor to spend time with them and I have learned much. I found things to emulate and things to avoid, inspiring examples and cautionary tales. Mostly I come away with stories that serve as "equipment for living," as Kenneth Burke put it. My encounters leave me with greater courage to live my own unfolding and uncertain story. I am less afraid of the future. I feel enlarged and more compassionate and often surprised by the joy and the sheer beauty of music, family, conversation, and nature.

Not long ago my daughter Emma gave birth to my grandson, Noah. I was reminded of a moving passage from Henri Nouwen's book *Aging: The Fulfillment of Life*. It describes an old wagon wheel leaning against a birch tree in the snow:

> The restful accomplishment of the old wheel tells us the story of life. Entering into the world we are what we are given, and for many years thereafter parents and grandparents, brothers and sisters, friends and lovers keep giving to us, some more, some less, some hesitantly, some generously. When we can finally stand on our own feet, speak our own words, and express our own unique self in work and love, we realize how much is given to us. But while reaching the height of our cycle, and saying with a great sense of confidence, "I really am," we sense that to fulfill our life we are now called to become parents and grandparents, brothers and sisters, teachers, friends, and lovers ourselves, and to give to others so that, when we leave this world, we can be what we have given.

What kind of old man will *I* be? How will I make a difference in other people's lives? How will I live a meaningful life in whatever physical body I inhabit? How will I continue to love and be loved?

Being an old man, I learned, can mean many things. Or it can mean nothing at all. When I began talking with these men, I thought that manhood was an important topic for everyone. I realize now that it was more important to me than it is to most of them. George Vaillant, scholar though he is of elite American manhood, identified more with his creativity than with his masculinity or sexuality. When I asked Dan Callahan what it meant to him to be an old man, he shrugged his shoulders. The question held no interest for him. Paul Volcker felt that he was less of a man, as did John Harper. Hugh Downs felt like less of a man physically and more of a man in other ways. Denton Cooley and Red Duke knew that they were men through and through, regardless of age.

As I began to lose my middle-aged strength, energy, and endurance in my early 60s, I often felt as if I were losing a piece of my manhood as well. It was emotionally difficult to walk on crutches, to be weak after surgery, or to spend days in bed. I wanted to feel like my usual strong and energetic self. In physical therapy after my first surgery, I was relieved when most of my strength came back. But no sooner did I feel like my usual self than another arthritic pain arose and then another surgery and then more physical therapy. Through it all, I have had the great good fortune of loving and being loved and cared for by Thelma Jean.

Today, when I see an old man bent over or limping, I do not see an Other. I see my future self. I watch Denton Cooley in a scooter. I walk behind Dan Callahan slowly shuffling up the stairs to his house. I listen to Sherwin Nuland's fear of being in a wheelchair. I know that my body will suffer more insults in the future, and that I will struggle emotionally. Yet I accept my vulnerability as part of being human. I do not feel that I am less of a man. When I reach the Fourth Age, I hope to answer the way Sam Karff did when I asked him what it was like to be an old man. "I feel old. I mean, I feel old," he said. "And I bear the name honorably. I don't pussyfoot and say seasoned or senior citizen. I'm an old man, and I'm very grateful to be an old man who is still functioning as well as I am."

I have worked as a humanities teacher, scholar, film maker, and ethics consultant in medical schools and colleges for more than 35 years. I am pleased with my external accomplishments. They made my mother proud and my university see that it was getting its money's worth out of me. But the most gratifying work has always been the quiet work of interacting with students, mentoring younger colleagues, working with older people in community settings, and interviewing people for films and books. It has been deeply gratifying to help students and others grow intellectually, personally and professionally—in small classrooms, one-on-one tutorials, or the informal mentoring that happens when they stop by. This might involve listening to private problems; witnessing the shock of students who saw their first patient die or who felt the joy of delivering their first baby; facilitating an open conversation among students or faculty; clearing a secure and confidential place for students to share difficult personal experiences as women, immigrants, persons of color, or followers of Islam; or leading writing workshops for older people whose lives were enlarged and shared. Interviewing men for *Old Man Country* created the same gratification for me and opened the same possibility of personal growth for them.

In a few years, I will step down from my job as Center Director. This will not be easy for me: What will I do? Who will I be? I want to feel less pressured by the demands of full-time work. I want to spend more time with Thelma Jean, to visit my children and to play with my grandson, to strengthen old friendships. And, like each of the men to whom I talked, I will still need to feel needed, to serve others, to feel that I am making a difference in the world. As Barbara Jordan, a Texas congresswoman in the 1970s, used to say, "You have to pay the rent for the space you occupy in life." I plan to pay the rent by working as a Spiritual Director and as an advocate for halting and reversing Climate Change.

But how will I matter if—more likely *when*—I become frail and dependent in the Fourth Age? How can old men still contribute as we decline and die? One way of contributing in the Fourth Age is to keep working to become our best selves. This might mean that we both resist and accept, even celebrate, the reality of our decline and dependence. Hugh Downs faces this paradox philosophically. While he exercises every day to maintain his muscle strength, he also accepts the inexorable biological process of senescence. "If you can't live with that you're going to be an unhappy person," he said to me. "But if you can, you realize that it is a beautiful thing that young people get older and that old people get older. That is nature."

Ram Dass takes the explicitly spiritual path of Hinduism, which demands a lifelong commitment to love, contemplation, and service. In spite of the debility and dependence that followed his devastating stroke, Ram Dass walks his own path toward merging with his view of ultimate reality. "I identify with my soul," he told me. The very real physical pain in his everyday life sometimes distracts him, but it does not overwhelm his capacity for fun and enjoyment along the way. And what about the quintessential Texan, Red Duke? In spite of back pain and a bum leg, he worked as a physician every day of his life until a broken heart valve put him in a wheelchair. At the end of his life, Duke's path took a form he learned as a boy hunting with his father. As he put it on his gravestone: *Piss on the fire. Call in the dogs. This hunt is over.*

James Forbes' life will always be framed by the words he heard while listening to Tchaikovsky in his dorm room at Howard University: *Jim Forbes, don't you know I am calling you? Jim Forbes, don't you know I am calling you?* John Harper will continue to find comfort and support in the various circles of his life. He will always be a member of the Episcopal Church, where he will minister to others and receive pastoral care himself. His gay friends form a family that will love and support him through the difficult passages ahead.

When I become frail, my existential significance will continue to be wrapped up with my family. I will still be a member of the covenant that God made with Noah and renewed with Abraham. I will still be a member of Temple Beth Israel in Houston and connected with Covenant Church, the small progressive Protestant church where I am welcomed as a Jew and have many strong friends. As a man who will be in the Fourth Age, I hope to wake up every day feeling grateful for being alive, for having my "soul restored to me in compassion," as the morning prayer puts it.

A week after new grandbaby Noah is born, I fly to Chicago to meet him and attend his bris, the Jewish ritual ceremony of circumcision. It is June 10, 2018, a chilly rainy morning. I take an Uber to see Emma and her husband Ben in their third-floor apartment near Wicker Park. Ben lets me inside. Soon after I sit down on the couch, Emma comes out of their bedroom and puts Noah in my arms.

"This is your grandson," she says.

I look at Noah, neatly swaddled and sleeping. A calm little miracle. "It's okay to cry, Dad," Emma says. "There's been a lot of crying around here."

In the book of Genesis, God tells Noah to build an ark of gopherwood and to bring inside his family and a male and a female from every species on earth. To punish humanity for its sins, God sends rain for 40 days and 40 nights, flooding the entire earth and destroying everything on it except Noah's ark. Rising waters lift the ark and send it adrift. After 40 days and 40 nights, the rain ceases. The water slowly subsides, and the ark settles down on the mountains of Ararat. God sets the moral terms of the covenant with Noah, who releases the animals and sets out with his family to establish civilization anew. Soon afterward, God paints a rainbow in the sky, a symbol of hope, a sign that God will never again destroy the world.

Before I leave Chicago and fly back to Houston, Ben takes a picture of me and Noah. In the picture, the outstretched fingers of my left hand reach toward Noah. His right hand reaches up, and four of his perfect tiny fingers curl around mine. We are holding onto each other for dear life.

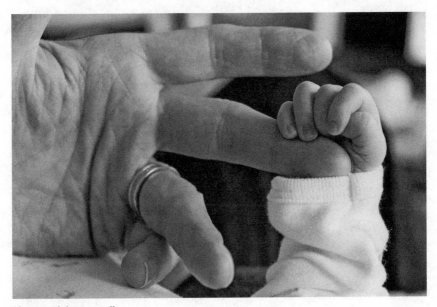

Photograph by Ben Hillson

## SOURCES AND FURTHER READING

Achenbaum, Andy. *Robert Butler, M.D.: Visionary of Healthy Aging*. New York: Columbia University Press, 2013.

Angell, Roger. *This Old Man*. New York: Doubleday, 2015.

Barnes, Julian. *Nothing to Be Afraid Of*. New York: Vintage, 2009.

Bialik, Hayyim Nahman, and Ravnitzky, Yehoshua, eds. *The Book of Legends/Sefer Ha-Aggadah: Legends from the Talmud and Midrash*. New York: Schocken, 1992.

Boutwell, Bryant. *I'm Dr. Red Duke*. College Station: Texas A&M Press, 2018.

Bunyan, John. *The Pilgrim's Progress*. New York: Signet, 2002. (Original work published 1678)

Butler, Robert. "Age-ism: Another Form of Bigotry." *The Gerontologist* 9, no. 4 (1969): 243–246.

Butler, Robert. *Why Survive? Being Old in America*. Baltimore: Johns Hopkins University Press, 1977.

Callahan, Daniel. *The Tyranny of Survival, and Other Pathologies of Civilized Life*. Bloomington: Indiana University Press, 1985.

Callahan, Daniel. *Setting Limits: Medical Goals in an Aging Society*. New York: Touchstone Books, 1988.

Callahan, Daniel. *Taming the Beloved Beast: Why Medical Technology Costs Are Destroying Our Health Care System*. Princeton, NJ: Princeton University Press, 2009.

Callahan, Daniel. *In Search of the Good: A Life in Bioethics*. Boston: MIT Press, 2012.

Callahan, Daniel. *The Five Horsemen of the Modern World: Climate Change, Food, Water, Disease, and Obesity*. New York: Columbia University Press, 2016.

Callahan, Sidney. "Abortion and the Sexual Agenda: A Case for Pro-Life Feminism." lib.tcu.edu/staff/bellinger/abortion/Callahan-Wolf.pdf

Cassidy, John. "The Volcker Rule." *The New Yorker*, July 26, 2010. Retrieved July 26, 2018, from https://www.newyorker.com/magazine/2010/07/26/the-volcker-rule

Coen, Joel, and Cohen, Ethan, directors. *No Country for Old Men* (DVD). Miramax Films, 2007.

Cole, Thomas R. *The Journey of Life: A Cultural History of Aging in America*. Cambridge, UK: Cambridge University Press, 1992.

Cole, Thomas R. *No Color Is My Kind: The Life of Eldrewey Stearns and the Integration of Houston.* Austin: University of Texas Press, 1997.

Cole, Thomas R., and Winkler, Mary, eds. *The Oxford Book of Aging.* Oxford, UK: Oxford University Press, 1994.

Cooley, Denton. *100,000 Hearts: A Surgeon's Memoir.* Austin: University of Texas Press, 2012.

Cowley, Malcolm. *The View from Eighty.* New York: Viking Press, 1980.

de Beauvoir, Simone. *La Vieillesse.* trans. by Patrick O'Brien as *The Coming of Age.* New York: Putnam, 1972.

deGrey, Aubrey. *Ending Aging.* New York: St. Martin's, 2007.

Downs, Hugh. *Thirty Dirty Lies About Old.* Boston: Hall, 1979.

Downs, Hugh. *Fifty to Forever.* Nashville, TN: Nelson, 1994.

Downs, Hugh. *Letter to a Great Grandson: A Message of Love, Advice, and Hopes for the Future.* Waterville, ME: Thorndike, 2005.

Eliot, T. S. "Four Quartets." Retrieved July 26, 2018, from http://www.davidgorman.com/4Quartets

Epstein, Joseph. "Review: The Art of Aging." *New York Times*, March 2, 2007. Retrieved July 26, 2018, from http://www.nytimes.com/2007/02/28/arts/28iht-idbriefs3A.4750568.html

Erikson, Erik. "Human Strength and the Cycle of Generations." In *Insight and Responsibility*, 109–158. New York: Norton, 1964.

Friedan, Betty. *The Fountain of Age.* London: Cape, 1993.

Forbes, James. *The Holy Spirit and Preaching.* Nashville, TN: Abingdon, 1989.

Forbes, James. *Whose Gospel? A Concise Guide to Progressive Preaching.* New York: New Press, 2010.

Gillick, Muriel. *The Denial of Aging: Perpetual Youth, Eternal Life, and Other Dangerous Fantasies.* Cambridge, MA: Harvard University Press, 2006.

Gillick, Muriel. *Old and Sick in America: The Journey Through the Health Care System.* Chapel Hill: University of North Carolina Press, 2017.

Gullette, Margaret. *Declining to Decline: Cultural Combat and the Politics of the Midlife.* Charlottesville: University Press of Virginia, 1997.

Gullette, Margaret. *Agewise: Fighting the New Ageism in America.* Chicago: University of Chicago Press, 2010.

Gullette, Margaret. *Ending Ageism or How Not to Shoot Old People.* New Brunswick, NJ: Rutgers University Press, 2017.

Hall, Donald. *Essays After 80.* New York: Mariner, 2014.

Hall, Donald. *A Carnival of Losses: Notes Nearing Ninety.* New York: Houghton Mifflin, 2018.

Hall, Stanley G. *Senescence: The Last Half of Life.* New York: Appleton, 1922.

Higgs, Paul, and Gilleard, Chris. *Rethinking Old Age: Theorizing the Fourth Age.* New York: Palgrave, 2010.

Holstein, Martha. *Women in Late Life: Critical Perspectives on Gender and Age.* London: Rowman & Littlefield, 2015.

Hudnut-Beumler, James, John W. Cook, Judith Weisenfeld, Leonora Tisdale, Lawrence Mamiya, and Peter J Paris. *The History of the Riverside Church in the City of New York.* New York: New York University Press, 2004.

Karff, Samuel. *Agada: The Language of Jewish Faith*. Brooklyn, NY: Ktav Publishing, 1979.

Karff, Samuel. *The Soul of the Rav: Sermons, Lectures, and Essays*. Woodway, TX: Eakin, 1999.

Karff, Samuel. *Permission to Believe: Finding Faith in Troubled Times*. Nashville, TN: Abingdon, 2005.

Karff, Samuel. *For This You Were Created: Memoir of an American Rabbi*. Houston, TX: Bright Sky Press, 2015.

Laslett, Peter. *A Fresh Map of Life: The Emergence of the Third Age*. Cambridge, MA: Harvard University Press, 1989.

Leland, John. *Happiness Is a Choice You Make: Lessons from a Year Among the Oldest Old*. New York: Farrar, Strauss & Giroux, 2017.

McCarthy, Cormac. *No Country for Old Men*. New York: Random House, 2005.

Moyers, Bill. "Speaking to Power: A NOW with Bill Moyers Special Edition." Retrieved July 26, 2018, from https://vimeo.com/127602087

Nouwen, Henri. *Aging: The Fulfillment of Life*. New York: Penguin, 1976.

Nuland, Sherwin B. *How We Die: Reflections on Life's Final Chapter*. New York: Vintage, 1993.

Nuland, Sherwin B. *Lost in America: A Journey with My Father*. New York: Vintage, 1993.

Nuland, Sherwin B. *The Art of Aging: A Doctor's Prescription for Well Being*. New York: Random House, 2007.

Palmer, Parker J. *On the Brink of Everything*. Oakland, CA: Berrett-Koehler, 2018.

Ram Dass. *Be Here Now*. San Cristobal, NM: Lama Foundation, 1971.

Ram Dass. *Journey of Awakening: A Meditator's Guidebook*. New York: Bantam, 1978.

Ram Dass. *Still Here: Embracing Aging, Changing and Dying*. New York: Riverhead, 2000.

Ram Dass. *Conversations with Ram Dass*. Los Angeles: Love Serve Remember Foundation, 2014.

Ram Dass, and Bush, Mirabai. *Compassion in Action: Setting out on the Path of Service*. New York: Bell Tower, 1985.

Ram Dass. *Fierce Grace* [documentary]. Directed by Mickey Lemly. New York: Zeitgeist Films, 2001.

Ram Dass. *Going Home* [film]. Directed by Derek Peck. Los Gatos, CA: Netflix, 2017.

Ram Dass, with Das, Rameshwar. *Be Love Now*. New York: HarperCollins, 2010.

Ram Dass, with Das, Rameshwar. *Polishing the Mirror: How to Live from Your Spiritual Heart*. Boulder, CO: Sounds True, 2013.

Rosin, Hannah. *The End of Men and the Rise of Women*. London: Penguin, 2012.

Schacter-Shalomi, Zalman, and Miller, Ronald S. *From Age-ing to Sage-ing: A Revolutionary Approach to Growing Older*. New York: Warner Books, 1997.

Shakespeare, William. *As You Like It*, edited by Juliet Dusinberre. London: Arden, 2006.

Shenk, Joshua Wolfe. "What Makes Us Happy?" *The Atlantic Magazine*, June 2009. Retrieved July 26, 2018, from https://www.theatlantic.com/magazine/archive/2009/06/what-makes-us-happy/307439

Small, Helen. *The Long Life*. Oxford, UK: Oxford University Press, 2007.

Specter-Mersel, Gabriella. "Never-Aging Stories: Western Hegemonic Masculinity Scripts." *Journal of Gender Studies* 15, no. 1 (2006): 67–82.

Thompson, Edward, Jr. *Older Men's Lives*. Thousand Oaks, CA: Sage, 1994.

Treaster, Joseph B. *Paul Volcker: The Making of a Financial Legend*. New York: Wiley, 2004.

Twigg, Julia, and Wendy Martin, eds. *Routledge Handbook of Cultural Gerontology*. New York: Routledge, 2015.

Vaillant, George. *The Natural History of Alcoholism*. Cambridge, MA: Harvard University Press, 1983.

Vaillant, George. *The Natural History of Alcoholism Revisited*. Cambridge, MA: Harvard University Press, 1995.

Vaillant, George. *Aging Well: Surprising Guideposts to a Happier Life from the Landmark Harvard Study of Adult Development*. Boston: Little, Brown, 2002.

Vaillant, George. *Spiritual Evolution: How We Are Wired for Faith, Hope, and Love*. New York: Broadway Books, 2008.

Vaillant, George. *Triumphs of Experience: The Men of the Harvard Grant Study*. Cambridge, MA: Belknap, 2012.

Vischer, A. L. *On Growing Old*. Translated by G. Onn. Boston: Houghton Mifflin, 1967.

Wink, Walter. *The Powers That Be: Theology for a New Millennium*. New York: Doubleday, 1998.

Wink, Walter. *Jesus and Nonviolence: A Third Way*. Minneapolis, MN: Fortress Press, 2003.

Wink, Walter. *Just Jesus: My Struggle to Become Human*. Syracuse, NY: Image, 2014.

Yeats, W. B. "Sailing to Byzantium." In *Selected Poems and Four Plays of William Butler Yeats*, edited by M. L. Rosenthal. New York: Scribner, 1996. (Original work published 1928)

*Interviews*

Edie Beaujon, November 8, 2016

Gene Buday, February 11, 2015

Dan Callahan, December 9, 2013

Dan and Sydney Callahan, December 29, 2016

Denton Cooley, September 29, 2015

Susan Cooley, March 20, 2018

Elizabeth Coulter, September 25, 2017

Hugh Downs, January 25, 2012

Red Duke, March 12, 2014

James Forbes, March 20, 2014

Stanislav Grof, July 7, 2016

Penelope Hall, September 8, 2017

Phil Hardberger, February 9, 2015

John Harper, July 24, 2017

Keith Jackson, September 29, 2015

Samuel Karff, March 29, 2013, and January 2, 2017

Robert Lane, September 27, 2016

Rick McCarthy, September 2017

Dee Morris, September 2017

Sherwin Nuland, March 12, 2014

Edmund Pellegrino, October 24, 2012

Ram Dass, September 28, 2017

William Schull, April 27, 2015

Rick Smith, June 12, 2015

George Vaillant, November 14, 2013

Paul Volcker, December 5, 2012

Walter Wink, February 18, 2011

# INDEX

*For the benefit of digital users, indexed terms that span two pages (e.g., 52–53) may, on occasion, appear on only one of those pages.*